Monograph Series in **Urology**

Volume 1

Endourology

Chief Editor

Arvind P Ganpule MS (Surgery), DNB (Urology), MNAMS (Urology)
Vice Chairman, Department of Urology
Chief, Division of Laparoscopic and Robotic Surgery
Muljibhai Patel Urological Hospital
Nadiad, Gujarat, India

Associate Editors

Abhishek Singh MS, MCh
Consultant Urologist
Muljibhai Patel Urological Hospital
Nadiad, Gujarat, India

V Mohan Kumar DNB, MRCS
Consultant Urologist
Muljibhai Patel Urological Hospital
Nadiad, Gujarat, India

Sudharsan Balaji MBBS, MS, MRCS, DNB
Consultant Urologist
Muljibhai Patel Urological Hospital
Nadiad, Gujarat, India

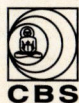

CBS

CBS Publishers & Distributors Pvt Ltd

New Delhi • Bengaluru • Chennai • Kochi • Kolkata • Mumbai
Bhopal • Bhubaneswar • Hyderabad • Jharkhand • Nagpur • Patna • Pune • Uttarakhand • Dhaka (Bangladesh)

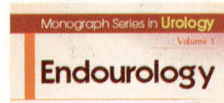

Monograph Series in **Urology**
Volume 1

Endourology

ISBN: 978-93-87964-13-6

First Edition: 2019

Published by Satish Kumar Jain and produced by Varun Jain for

CBS Publishers & Distributors Pvt Ltd
4819/XI Prahlad Street, 24 Ansari Road, Daryaganj, New Delhi 110 002, India.
Ph: 23289259, 23266861, 23266867   Fax: 011-23243014   Website: www.cbspd.com
                                                                                        e-mail: delhi@cbspd.com; cbspubs@airtelmail.in
Corporate Office: 204 FIE, Industrial Area, Patparganj, Delhi 110 092
Ph: 4934 4934   Fax: 4934 4935   e-mail: publishing@cbspd.com; publicity@cbspd.com

Branches

- **Bengaluru:** Seema House 2975, 17th Cross, K.R. Road,
  Banasankari 2nd Stage, Bengaluru 560 070, Karnataka
  Ph: +91-80-26771678/79   Fax: +91-80-26771680   e-mail: bangalore@cbspd.com
- **Chennai:** 7, Subbaraya Street, Shenoy Nagar, Chennai 600 030, Tamil Nadu
  Ph: +91-44-26680620, 26681266   Fax: +91-44-42032115   e-mail: chennai@cbspd.com
- **Kochi:** 42/1325, 1326, Power House Road, Opposite KSEB Power House,
  Ernakulam 682 018, Kochi, Kerala
  Ph: +91-484-4059061-65   Fax: +91-484-4059065   e-mail: kochi@cbspd.com
- **Kolkata:** 6/B, Ground Floor, Rameswar Shaw Road, Kolkata-700 014, West Bengal
  Ph: +91-33-22891126, 22891127, 22891128   e-mail: kolkata@cbspd.com
- **Mumbai:** 83-C, Dr E Moses Road, Worli, Mumbai-400018, Maharashtra
  Ph: +91-22-24902340/41   Fax: +91-22-24902342   e-mail: mumbai@cbspd.com

Representatives

• Bhopal	0-8319310552	• Bhubaneswar	0-9911037372	• Hyderabad	0-9885175004	• Jharkhand	0-9811541605
• Nagpur	0-9021734563	• Patna	0-9334159340	• Pune	0-9623451994	• Uttarakhand	0-9716462459
• Dhaka (Bangladesh)	01912-003485						

Printed at Paras Offset Pvt. Ltd., New Delhi, India

to

---

our teachers for, without them,
we could not have been where we are now...

our family members for their time and
who have been patient throughout the creation of this book...

And, last but not the least, our patients without whom we could not have
acquired anything, neither knowledge nor the skill...

Monograph Series in Urology

Volume 1

Endourology

Contributors

Amit Bhattu
Consultant Urologist
Jupiter Hospitals
Thane, Maharashtra, India
Section 2: RIRS

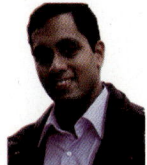

Rajesh Kukreja
Consultant Urologist
Urocare Clinic, Indore, Madhya Pradesh
Section 1: PCNL

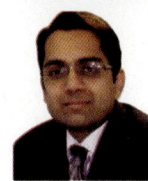

Sudharsan Balaji
Consultant Urologist
Muljibhai Patel Urological Hospital
Dr Virendra Desai Road, Nadiad, India
Section 2: RIRS

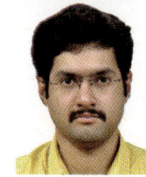

Foreword

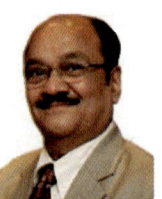

I have witnessed over the past four decades of my career as an urologist that "In science nothing is constant, change is the rule". It was in the eighth decade of the last century that urology as a specialty diversified from its parent organization, the Association of Surgeons of India (ASI). In next two decades urology community witnessed an explosion of technology and technique which was responsible for urology to grow in leaps and bounds. The ulitimate beneficiaries were the patients. As the story progresses, we now stand in 2018 with subspecialization the rule and not the exception. The future of urology is subspecialization.

Urology, as the specialty is blessed to have a plethora of subspecialty ranging from urooncology to female urology, robotics and laparoscopy included. Dr Arvind P Ganpule and his illustrious team of authors, who I am proud to note are my students, have compiled an impressive series of monographs. The monograph series gets well the future of subspecialization in urology.

In Volume 1, the authors have gone back to the basics of endourology. I have no doubt that this volume would be considered in the future as a reference text for students of the art of endourology. Volume 2 is the heart of the series. As it was said famously "laparoscopic surgery stands on the shoulders of open surgery while robotic surgery stands on the able shoulders of laparoscopic surgery". Volume 2 exactly achieves the goal of this quote as it dwells on the basic principles in laparoscopic urology which includes ergonomics, instrumentation and port placements in laparoscopic nephrectomy, laparoscopic pyeloplasty and laparoscopic adrenalectomies. Last but not the least, the Volume 3 includes important considerations in robotic/laparoscopic surgeries and vascular reconstructions.

I am sure this series of monographs on important urology topics will go a long way in educating medical students, urology residents and urologists alike.

Mahesh Desai MS, FRCS
Managing Trustee, Muljibhai Patel Urological Hospital, Nadiad, India
Past Medical Director, Muljibhai Patel Urological Hospital, Nadiad, India
Past Chairman, Department of Urology, Muljibhai Patel Urological Hospital, Nadiad
Past President, Urological Society of India (USI), Endourological Society
Societe Internationale de Urologie (SIU)

Foreword

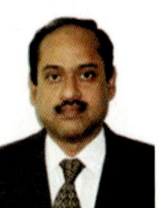

Urology is a superspecialty, which is rapidly advancing. New procedures, imaging modalities, instruments and energy sources have come in last 5–10 years, which have changed the way we look at urology. Several methods which were treatment of choice a decade ago, now have become obsolete. Naturally, it is a challenge to remain updated with all such advances. Quite often, textbooks give so much information about everything that specific details about particular thing lack or difficult to search. Hence, if reader wants to find out details and nuances, he has to refer to journals or books dedicated to that topic. Monographs are extremely useful in such situations.

Dr Ganpule and his team of authors have specifically addressed this problem and have come out with monographs on various topics. Monographs generally become popular and are liked by many, because all details they obtain from it. Endourology and laparoscopy are the areas where maximum advances have happened and will happen in the future and I am happy that Dr Ganpule has dedicated first and second volumes to these areas giving all details from basic to advances, technical details and troubleshooting. Third volume is addressed to miscellaneous areas which generally are not covered in detail in other reference textbooks.

Although there are three volumes, readers have option to buy any volume as per their areas of interest. These monograph volumes are particularly useful to residents and junior consultants. Troubleshooting will be very useful to overcome any problems they face in their practice.

I must congratulate Dr Ganpule and all the contributors for putting huge efforts and compiling all details in the form of monographs in three exhaustive volumes.

Ravindra B Sabnis MS, MCh
Honorary Secretary
Urological Society of India
Chairman, Department of Urology
Muljibhai Patel Urological Hospital
Nadiad, Gujarat, India

Preface

The idea of this series of monographs was realized while attending one of the theme-based conferences. As we move towards theme-based meetings from large congresses, continuing medical education programmes and conferences, we thought of having a series of informative booklets on selected topics. Basically these should be topics which are tailored for selected audience. The urological world is moving towards subspecialization. Given this paradigm shift, we are witnessing over the past decade, this monograph series is timely, apts and addresses all the requirements of the hour.

Myself along with Mr Ramesh of CBS Publishers & Distributors, Mumbai, have aimed to come out with a collection of monographs (would be available as a basket/bunch of monographs) in urology.

Another intent of coming out with this project is to provide postgraduates, young consultants and practicing urologists, a compilation which describes common urological procedures in the format of colour atlas, bail me out! Tips and finally a review of contemporary literature. We would be emphasizing on the techniques of the procedure.

The series comprises monographs in endourology, laparoscopy and short monographs on practical tips in urology. Each of these monographs focuses on technical aspects on the subject, troubleshooting and the relevant literature on the subject.

The topics range from basics in laparoscopy and robotics to nitty gritties in vascular reconstruction.

Needless to say, all the bouquets of compliments should be reserved for the authors and the contributors and brickbats and critiques for me. I hope, this academic endeavor will provide a useful read and achieve its goals.

Last but not the least, if it was not the enthusiasm and initiative of Mr Ramesh, this monograph series would not have been a reality. Any academic initiative is not possible without the support of residents. I acknowledge my gratitude towards them. A big thanks to CBS Publishers & Distributors, Mr SK Jain CMD, and Mr YN Arjuna Senior Vice President—Publishing, Editorial and Publicity, Mrs Ritu Chawla General Manager—Production, Mr Vikrant Sharma, Mr Sanjay Chauhan and Mr Ananda Mohanty apart from the great support staff at their easily accessible office. I would like to acknowledge the support of my associate editors who made sure that this project sees the light of the day.

Arvind P Ganpule
Nadiad, India

Contents

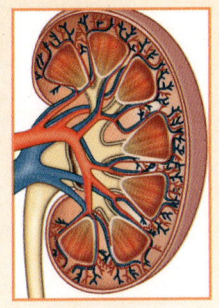

Section

I

Percutaneous Nephrolithotomy (PCNL)

Rajesh Kukreja

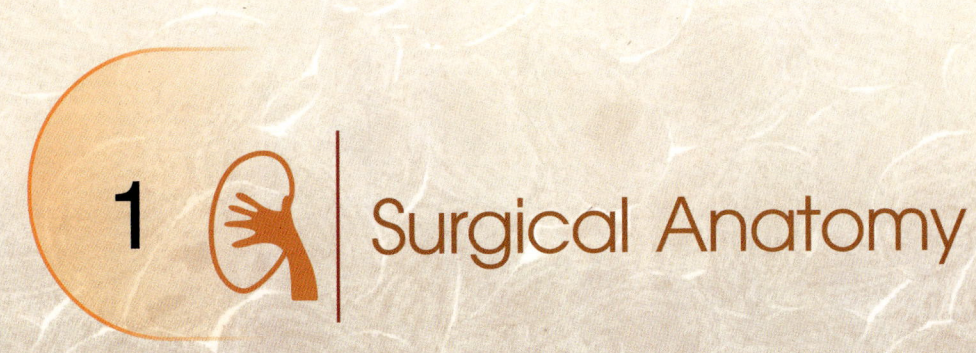

Rajesh Kukreja

The visualization of the kidney and surrounding structures during standard percutaneous entry guided by fluoroscopy or ultrasonography is limited. Understanding of the renal and perirenal anatomy is critical for obtaining access that is both effective and safe. Even armed with this knowledge, variations in anatomy can make access challenging for the experienced surgeon and prohibitive for the inexperienced done.[1]

The Three 30 Degrees

The kidneys lie on the posterior abdominal wall against the psoas muscle.

- The longitudinal axis of the kidneys parallels the lateral edges of the psoas muscles, about 30 degrees from vertical, with the lower poles lateral to the upper poles (Fig. 1.1A to F).
- Due to the cone shaped psoas major muscle, the kidneys are also tilted 30 degrees off the frontal plane, with the lower poles anterior to the upper poles (Fig. 1.1B).
- Finally, the kidneys are rotated out of the frontal plane as well due to the psoas muscle, with the lateral aspect of the kidney posterior to the medial aspect, such that each kidney is rotated 30 degrees posteriorly from the renal hilum (Fig. 1.1C).[1]

In prone position, the pelvis tends to fall anteriorly on the psoas muscle; hence the lower pole, pelvis and the proximal end of the ureter are placed more anteriorly than the upper pole.

The Renal Coverings

The kidney surface is enclosed in a continuous covering of fibrous tissue, the renal capsule ("true renal capsule"). Each kidney within its capsule is surrounded by a mass of adipose tissue, lying between the peritoneum and the posterior abdominal wall. This perirenal fat is enclosed by the renal fascia (the so-called fibrous renal fascia of Gerota). The renal fascia is enclosed anteriorly and posteriorly by another layer of adipose tissue, the pararenal fat, which varies in thickness. The renal fascia is made up of a posterior layer (a well defined and strong structure) and an anterior layer (a more delicate structure, which tends to adhere to the peritoneum). The anterior and posterior layers of the renal fascia (fascia of Gerota) subdivide the retroperitoneal space into three potential compartments: (1) the posterior pararenal space (P), which contains only fat; (2) the intermediate perirenal space (I), which contains the suprarenal glands, kidneys and proximal ureters, together with the perirenal fat; and (3) the anterior pararenal space (A), which unlike the posterior and intermediate spaces, extends across the midline from one side of the abdomen to the other. This latter space contains the

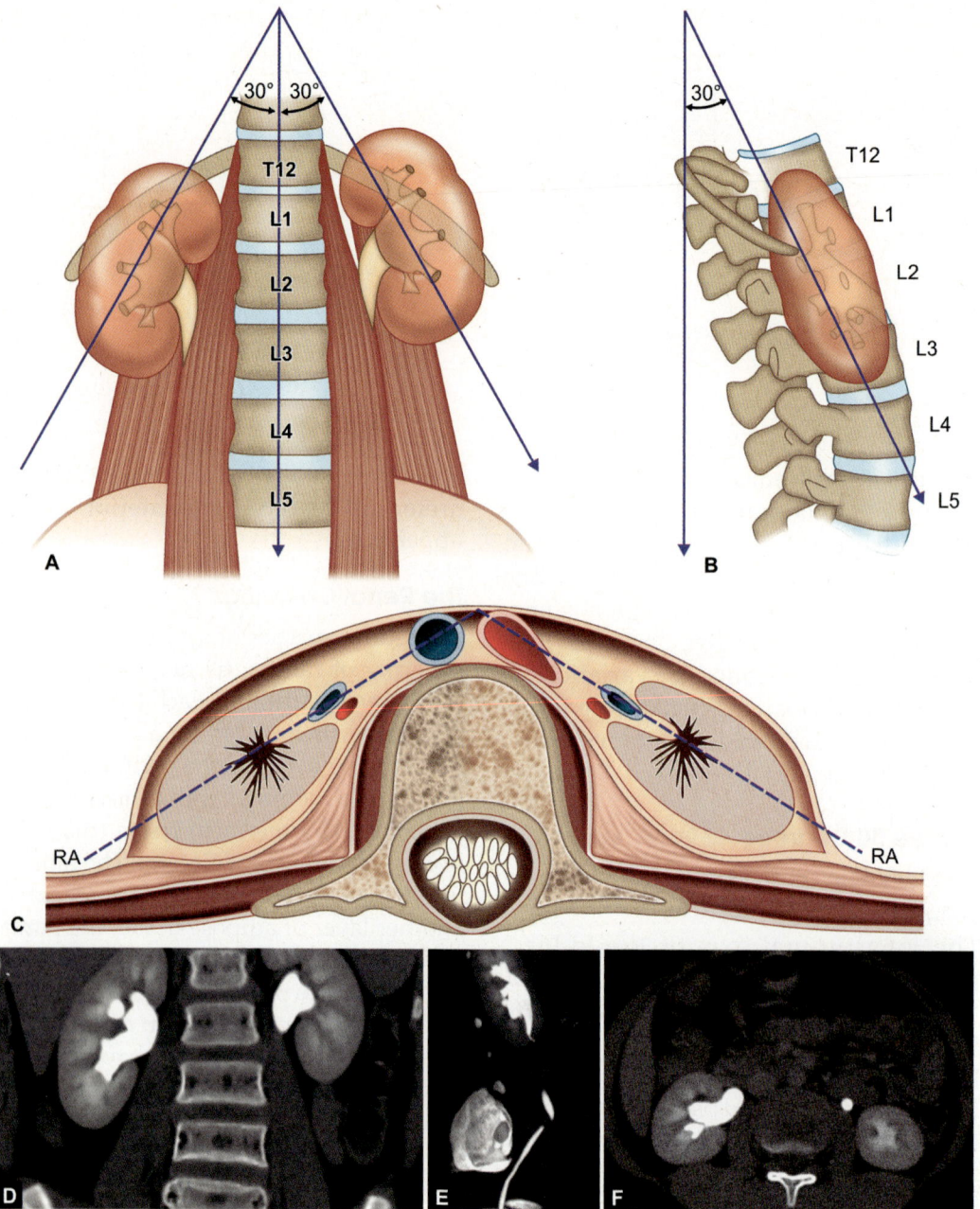

Fig. 1.1A to F: The three 30 degrees

ascending and descending colon, the duodenal loop and the pancreas.

Inferiorly, the layers of the renal fascia end weakly fused around the ureter. Superiorly, the two layers of the renal fascia fuse above the suprarenal gland and end fused with the infradiaphragmatic fascia. An additional fascial layer separates the suprarenal gland from the kidney. Laterally, the two layers of the renal fascia fuse behind the ascending and descending colons. Medially, the posterior fascial layer is fused with the fascia of the spine muscles. The anterior fascial layer merges into the connective tissue of the great vessels (aorta and inferior vena cava). These anatomic descriptions of the renal fascia show that the right and left perirenal spaces are potentially separated and, therefore, it is exceptional that a complication of an endourologic procedure, e.g. hematoma, urinoma, or perirenal abscess, involves the contralateral perirenal space (Fig. 1.2).[2]

The Calyceal Anatomy

The renal papillae drain into the minor calyces, which are the most peripheral portions of the intrarenal collecting system. If only one papilla drains into a minor calyx, it is described as a simple calyx. When there are two or more papillae entering the calyx, it is termed a compound calyx. The outermost wall of the calyx, into which the papilla is set, is the calyceal fornix. There are 5 to 14 minor calyces

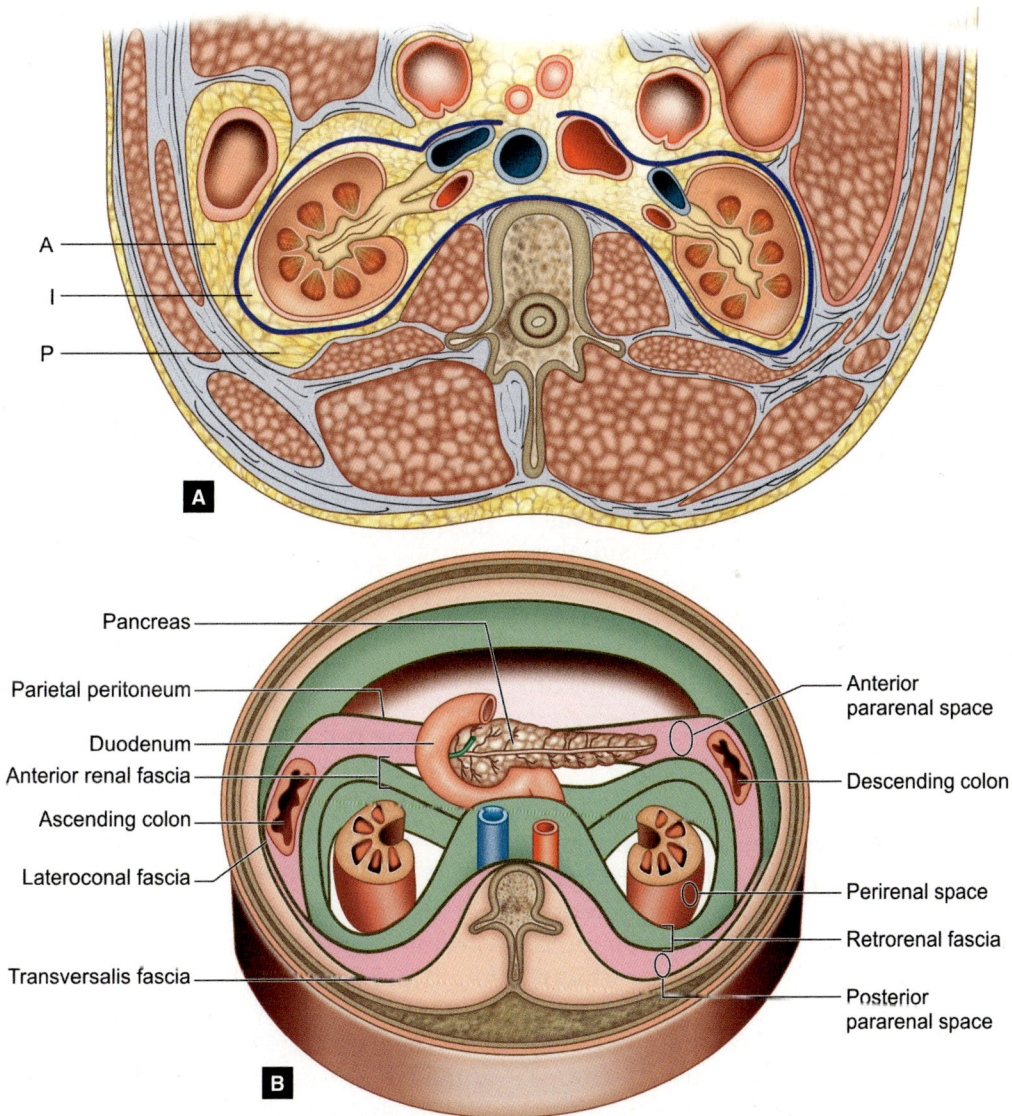

A
I
P

A

Pancreas
Parietal peritoneum
Duodenum
Anterior renal fascia
Ascending colon
Lateroconal fascia
Transversalis fascia

Anterior pararenal space
Descending colon
Perirenal space
Retrorenal fascia
Posterior pararenal space

B

Fig. 1.2A and B: The renal coverings

in each kidney (mean of 8, with 70% of kidneys having 7 to 9 minor calyces).[3] There are three calyceal groups: The upper, middle and lower. Compound calyces are the rule in the upper calyceal group, are common in the lower calyceal group, and are rare in the middle calyceal group. The minor calyces, either directly or after coalescing into major calyces, drain by infundibula into the renal pelvis. Occasionally, a minor calyx will open directly into the renal pelvis without an intervening infundibulum. Some infundibula are unusually narrow, even if they drain adequately, and they can present an obstacle to endoscopy, especially with the relatively large rigid nephroscope.[1]

Sampaio found that, in the cases he studied, the superior pole was drained by only one midline calyceal infundibulum in 98.6% of cases; the inferior pole was drained by paired calyces arranged in two rows in 58% and by a single midline calyceal infundibulum in 42% of cases and the mid-pole was drained by paired calyces arranged in two rows (anterior and posterior) in 96% of cases.[2-4] This has important implications for percutaneous renal access as it will be easier to access endoscopically a polar region drained by a single infundibulum, which usually has suitable diameter, rather than a polar region drained by paired calyces. He also found that, for best access to the pelvic-ureteric junction (PUJ), one should choose a pole whose calyx forms an angle of 90° or more with the PUJ.

Classification of the Pelvicalyceal System[2]

The analysis of 140 endocasts led Sampaio to a division into two major groups (with two intermediate varieties in each major group). This division was based on superior pole, inferior pole and kidney midzone (hilar) calyceal drainage.

Group A is composed of pelvicalyceal systems that have two major calyceal groups (superior and inferior) as a primary division of the renal pelvis and a midzone calyceal drainage dependent on these two major groups (62.2%). It includes two different types of pelvicalyceal system:

- Type A-I (45%). The kidney midzone is drained by minor calyces that are dependent on the superior and/or inferior calyceal groups.
- Type A-II (17.2%). The kidney midzone is drained simultaneously by crossed calyces, one draining into the superior calyceal group and the other draining into the inferior calyceal group. The crossed calyces (laterally) and the renal pelvis (medially) bound a region (space) that is designated the "interpelvicalyceal" (IPC) region (space). Detection of an interpelvicalyceal (IPC) region on the pyelogram is an indirect sign of crossed calyces in the kidney midzone. When the crossed calyces were in the midkidney, the calyx draining into the inferior calyceal group was in the ventral position in 87.5% of the endocasts.

Group B is composed of pelvicalyceal systems with kidney midzone (hilar) calyceal drainage independent of both the superior and inferior calyceal groups (37.8%). This group also includes two different types of pelvicalyceal systems:

- Type B-I (21.4%). The kidney midzone is drained by a major calyceal group, independent of both the superior and the inferior groups.
- Type B-II (16.4%). The kidney midzone is drained by minor calyces (one to four) entering directly into the renal pelvis. Such calyces are independent of both the superior and inferior calyceal groups.

The kidney collecting system is very variable and is not symmetrical. Sampaio found pelvicalyceal systems with morphologic bilateral symmetry in the same individual in only 37.1% of the cases. In 11.4% of the endocasts, there was a perpendicular minor calyx draining directly into the renal pelvis or into a major calyx. Stones in such minor calyces viewed on standard antero-posterior radiographic images can appear as if they were placed in the pelvis or a major calyx. Thus, this anatomic detail must be considered in cases of stones that do not alter renal function and can appear as if they are in the renal pelvis or a major calyx. In this situation, a complementary radiologic study with lateral and oblique films must be performed to determine accurately the position and extent of the stones. When a stone is located in a perpendicular minor calyx, its removal presents additional difficulties for percutaneous nephrolithotomy (PCNL). Direct access into the calyx containing the stone is easy; nevertheless, it involves a puncture without consideration of the arterial and venous anatomic relationships to the collecting system, which carries a high risk of injuring a vascular structure. Therefore, in cases of stone in such calyces, safe access, techniques and instruments should be used.

Identifying the Posterior Calyx: The Big Dilemma

An important consideration for percutaneous renal surgery is the determination of the anteroposterior orientation of the calyces, because access (from the typical posterior or posterolateral approach) into a posterior calyx allows relatively straight entry into the rest of the kidney, whereas percutaneous puncture of an anterior calyx requires an acute angulation to enter the renal pelvis, which may not be possible with rigid instrumentation.

Investigators have attempted to differentiate calyces as anterior or posterior solely on the basis of their medial or lateral orientation as seen on IVU. The available anatomical references on this aspect are contradictory, confusing and incomplete. In 1901, Brodel studied corrosion casts of 70 cadaveric kidneys. He depicted the anterior calyces as medial and posterior as lateral. Hodson, in 1972, described exactly the opposite, i.e. the anterior calyces located laterally and posterior

calyces located medially. Then, in 1984, Kaye and Reinke measured calyceal angles from the axial CT images. They concluded that the Brodel pattern is seen in 69% of right kidneys while 70% of left kidneys have a Hodson pattern.

Sampaio et al studied 140 endocasts and found that the anterior calyces are lateral in 28%, posterior calyces are lateral in 19%, and in 53% endocasts the anterior and posterior calyces had varied positions, superimposed or alternately distributed. He found that the calyceal orientation was region dependent. The typical anterior and posterior pattern of the calyces is seen only in the middle pole. The lower pole has this arrangement in only 58% cases while the upper pole almost uniformly has a compound calyceal system. This implies that in the lower and upper pole the calyces are dominantly oriented in the direction of their respective poles.

Miller studied detailed renal calyceal anatomy obtained from *in vivo* three-dimensional computerized tomography (CT) renderings.[5] The primary plane of the upper pole calyceal group was mediolateral (ML) in 95% of kidneys and a combination of antero-posterior (AP) and ML in 5%. The middle calyceal group had a primary plane of AP in 100% of kidneys. The primary plane of the lower pole calyceal group was AP in 95% of kidneys, ML in 3% and a combination of AP and ML in 2%.

Computerized tomography (CT) reconstruction and assessment preoperatively helps in defining the calyceal anatomy and planning the calyceal entry (Fig. 1.3). A well-studied IVU also helps in near accurate estimation of the posterior calyx (Fig. 1.4).

Upper Polar Access

Miller et al found that in the upper pole, the primary plane of the calyces in the upper pole was medial/lateral and generally neutral relative to the anteroposterior (AP) axis of the kidney. As the upper pole is more posterior in the prone position, access via any calyx would provide a working tract that parallels

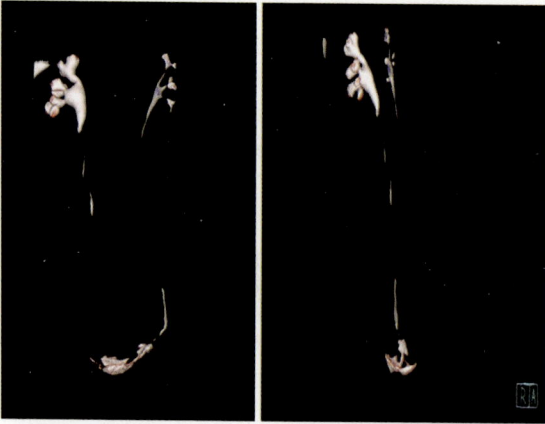

Fig. 1.3: Reconstruction: Anteroposterior (AP) and oblique views help identifying the posterior calyces

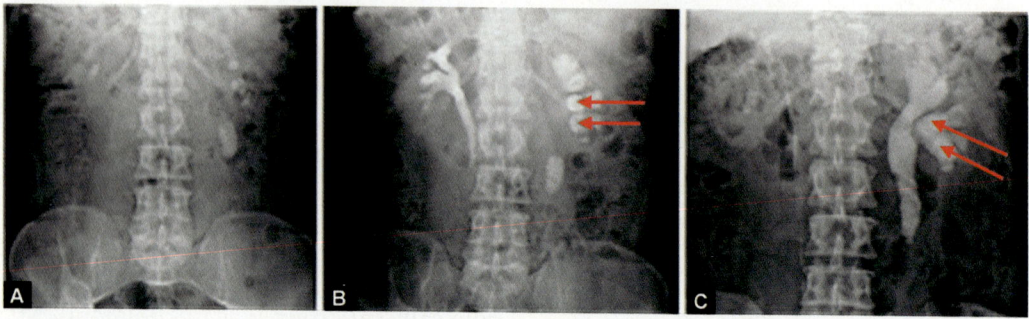

Fig. 1.4: Red arrows indicate posterior calyces. (A) Plain X-ray KUB; (B) IVP (supine, 10 min): Posterior calyces fill up early; (C) IVP (prone, delayed): Posterior calyces are overlapped by dye in infundibula and anterior calyces

the longitudinal axis of the kidney. This would mean access via an angle which would allow rigid instruments to reach most of the calyces in the kidney. However, preferably the lateral most calyx should be punctured in the upper pole as puncturing a medial calyx is associated with significant risk of causing injury to the posterior segmental artery and puncturing the pleura.

Lower Polar Access

CT scans were analyzed for 101 renal units (50 left; 51 right) by Eisner and Stoller.[6] For the lower pole, 42 (41.6%) renal unit shad two calyces and 59 (58.4%) renal units had three calyces. The most medial calyx on two-dimensional imaging, the first calyx, is almost always anterior facing and the most anterior lower-pole calyx, therefore, it is suboptimal for lower pole percutaneous renal access. The calyx just lateral to the medial calyx, the second calyx, is statistically the most likely to be posterior facing and the most posterior positioned calyx and should be targeted for percutaneous lower-pole renal puncture to ensure optimal access to the collecting system (Fig. 1.5).

Intrarenal Vasculature

The safest place to access percutaneously, the collecting system is directly into the calyceal fornix, because this will avoid the interlobar (infundibular) arteries adjacent to the calyceal infundibula and the arcuate arteries that skirt the renal pyramid.

The short renal hilar vessels limit the mobility of the kidneys, although nephroptosis

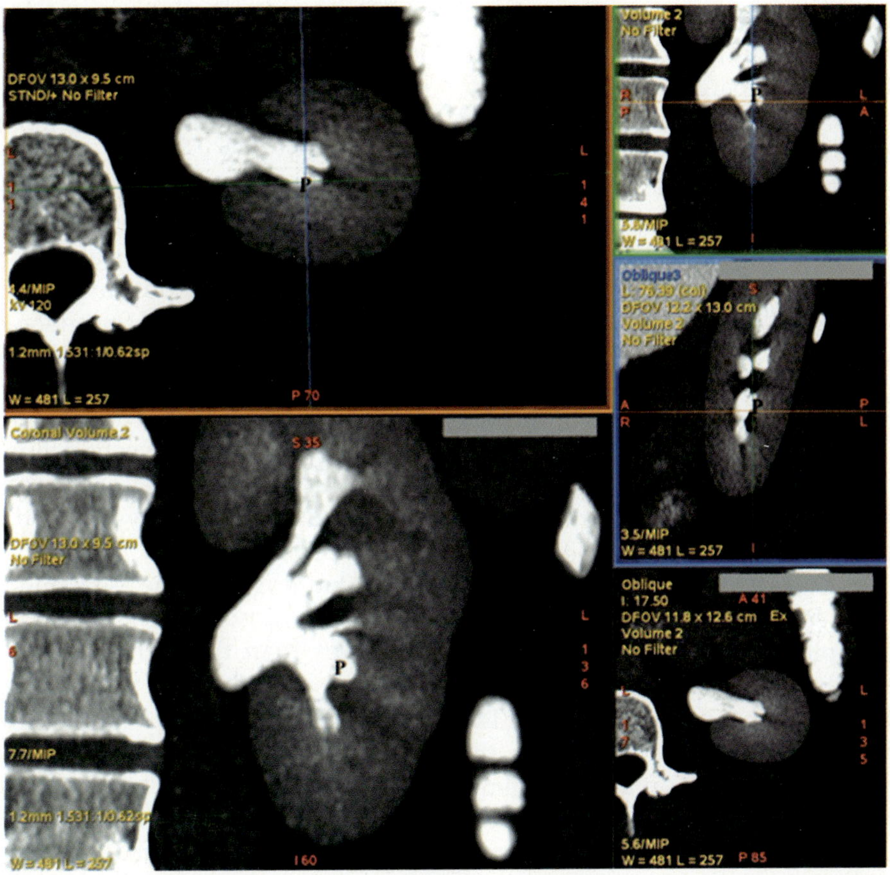

Fig. 1.5: Identifying the lower posterior calyx: CT images in coronal, axial and sagittal planes help identify the posterior lower calyx (indicated in all images as "P" at intersection of horizontal and vertical cursor lines

("falling kidney") can occur, especially in thin women with a paucity of perirenal fat. In such cases, the kidney not only descends but also rotates anteriorly. This can be troublesome during percutaneous punctures with the patient in a prone position.

The main renal artery divides into an anterior and a posterior branch. The former then divides within or before the renal sinus into four anterior segmental arteries: The apical and lower segmental arteries (which supply the tip of the upper pole and the entire lower pole, respectively), and the upper and middle segmental arteries (which supply the remainder of the anterior half of the kidney) (Fig. 1.6). The posterior branch of the renal artery supplies the remainder of the posterior

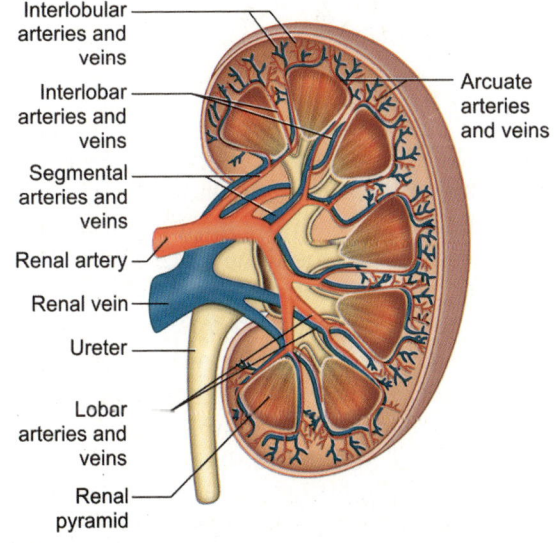

Interlobular arteries and veins

Interlobar arteries and veins

Segmental arteries and veins

Renal artery

Renal vein

Ureter

Lobar arteries and veins

Renal pyramid

Arcuate arteries and veins

Fig. 1.6: The intrarenal vasculature

half of the kidney. After the anterior segmental arteries and the posterior branch of the renal artery enter the renal parenchyma, they divide into interlobar arteries, which are also called infundibular arteries owing to their course adjacent to the calyceal infundibula of the renal collecting system. At the cortico-medullary junction, near the base of the renal pyramids, each interlobar artery usually divides into two arcuate arteries that run along the renal pyramid. The next division is into the interlobular arteries, which run along the outer surface of the renal pyramids and are derived at right angles from the arcuate arteries. The final divisions, the afferent arterioles of the glomeruli, come off the interlobular arteries in the peripheral renal cortex. Each renal arteriole is an "end-artery", meaning that each cell in the kidney derives its blood supply from one arteriole. For this reason renal arterial vascular injury must be avoided to prevent loss of renal function. The potential for arterial injury is least in the Brödel line, which is an avascular plane approximately at the lateral margin of the kidney (Figs 1.7 and 1.8), extending from the superior apex of the kidney (limited by the circulation of the apical anterior segmental artery) to the lower pole of the kidney (limited by the circulation of the lower anterior segmental artery).

Regional Vascular Anatomy of the Kidney

Sampaio analyzed 82, 3D polyester resin corrosion endocasts of the kidney collecting system together with the intrarenal arteries, and 52 endocasts of the kidney collecting system together with the intrarenal veins, obtained according to the injection-corrosion technique.

Puncture is most dangerous through the upper pole infundibulum because this region is surrounded almost completely by large vessels (Table 1.1). Infundibular arteries and veins course parallel to the anterior and posterior aspects of the upper pole infundi-bulum. Injury to an interlobar (infundibular) vessel was a common consequence of puncturing the upper pole infundibulum (67% of kidneys); the injured vessel was an artery in 26% of those cases. The most serious vascular accident in upper infundibulum puncture is lesion of the posterior segmental artery (retropelvic artery). This event may occur because this artery was crossed by and is related to the posterior surface of the upper infundibulum in 57% of the endocasts.

In the inferior pole, a collar-like venous anastomosis around the minor calyces infundibula (calyceal necks) is often found. Puncture through the lower pole infundibulum, therefore, also risks injury to a venous arcade.[2]

Relationship of kidneys to the diaphragm, ribs and pleura.

The kidneys lie on the psoas and quadratus lumborum muscles. Usually, the left kidney is higher than the right kidney, with the posterior surface of the right kidney crossed by the 12th rib and the left kidney crossed by the 11th and 12th ribs. The posterior surface of the diaphragm attaches to the extremities of the 11th and 12th ribs. Close to the spine, the diaphragm is attached over the posterior abdominal muscles, and forms the medial and lateral arcuate ligaments on each side. In this way, the posterior aspect of the diaphragm (posterior leaves) arches in a dome above the superior pole of the kidneys, on each side. Therefore, when performing an intrarenal access by puncture, the endourologist may consider that the diaphragm is traversed by all intercostal punctures, and possibly by some punctures below the 12th rib.

Stening and Bourne have discussed in depth the anatomic considerations in the supracostal approach for renal surgery.[7] The lower limit of the parietal pleura crosses the 12th rib obliquely at its midpoint such that the lateral half of the rib is uncovered by the pleura. In the midscapular line, the visceral pleura is in relation to the 10th rib, while the parietal pleura is at the level of the 12th rib. The parietal and visceral pleura ascend cranially and laterally on the ribs, and further

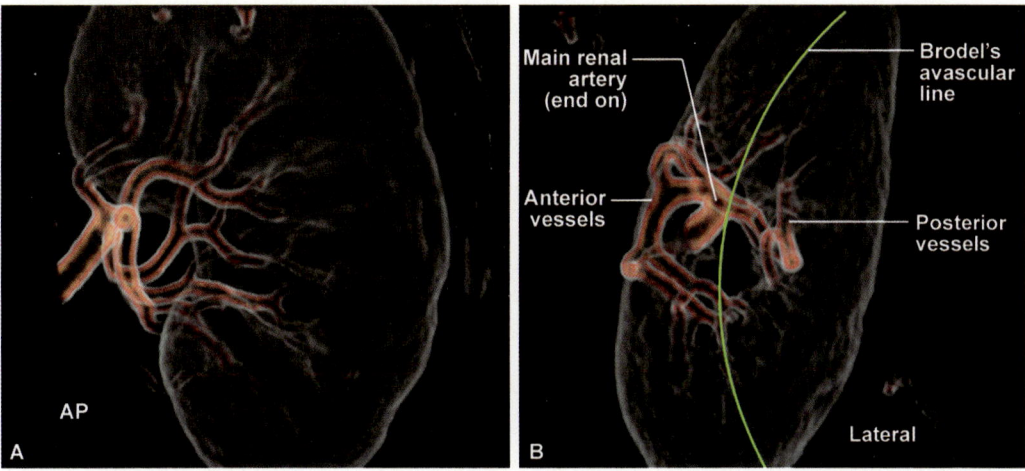

Fig. 1.7: CT angiogram reconstruction showing intrarenal vasculature. A: Anteroposterior view; B: Lateral view

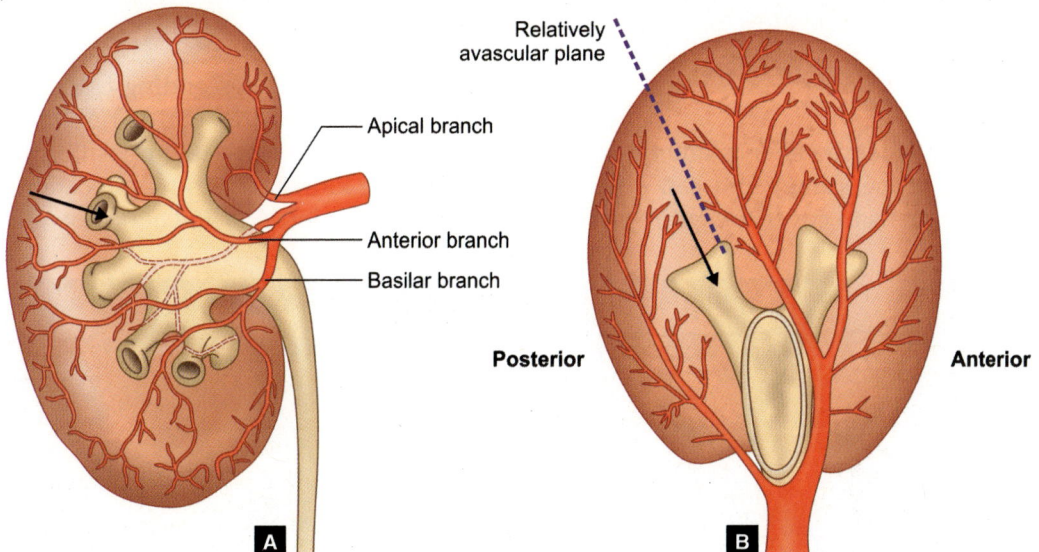

Fig. 1.8: Relatively avascular areas for proper renal calyceal puncture. (A) Coronal view: Between and parallel to interlobar arteries; (B) Axial view: Along the Brodel line between the anterior and posterior circulation

Table 1.1: Relation of the infundibula with major vessels[2]			
Infundibuli	*Vessels*	*Presence of artery (%)*	*Presence of vein (%)*
Upper	Interlobar/Segmental	86.6	84.6
Middle anteriorly	Interlobar/Segmental	65	71
Middle posteriorly	Mid-subdivision branch of the posterior segmental artery (retropelvic artery)	100	21
Lower anteriorly	Inferior segmental	100	100
Lower posteriorly	Extension of posterior segmental artery	38	21

rise in deep expiration (Figs 1.9 and 1.10). Thus, a puncture made lateral to the midscapular line, below the 10th rib, in deep expiration would almost always prevent damage to the visceral pleura. Tracts below the 11th rib made lateral to the midscapular line would miss not only the visceral pleura but also may miss the parietal pleura (Figs 1.9C and 1.10C). Tracts made through the parietal pleura may not be of clinical significance, especially when the Amplatz sheath is used, because this would avoid the leakage of the irrigation fluid in the pleural space by maintaining a low-pressure irrigation. Any intercostal puncture should be made in the lower half of the intercostal space, in order to avoid injury to the intercostal vessels above.

Relationship of Kidneys to the Liver and Spleen

On the right side, the liver is anterior to the upper pole of the kidney and can extend in some individuals to cover the entire anterior surface. On the left, the spleen covers less of the kidney anteriorly. Both the liver and spleen can extend lateral to the kidneys and are therefore at risk of injury with a lateral puncture into the kidney (Fig. 1.11). The liver on the right side and the spleen on the left may be posterolaterally positioned at the level of the suprahilar region of the kidney, because at this point these organs have their largest dimensions. If the intrarenal puncture is performed when the patient is in mid or full inspiration, the risk of injury to the liver and spleen is increased. This knowledge is particularly important in patients with hepatomegaly or splenomegaly, in whom a CT scan should be performed before puncturing the kidney.

The Colon

The ascending and descending colon can be lateral or even posterior to the right and left kidneys, respectively. The opposition of the colon to the kidney varies with location; it is greatest on the left side and at the lower pole.

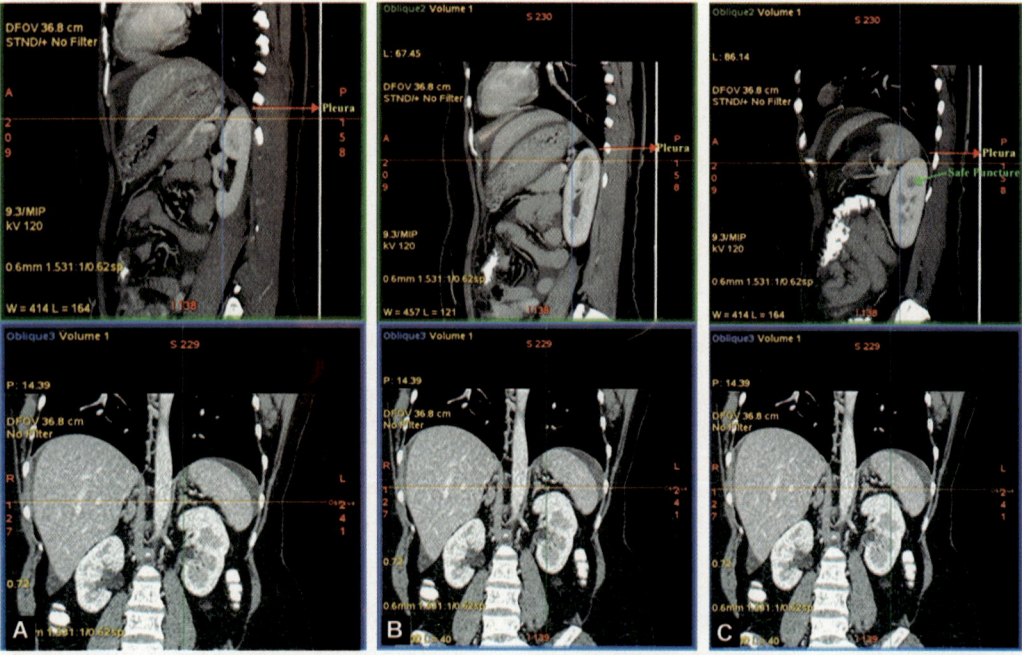

Fig. 1.9: Relationship of pleura with the upper pole of kidney during inspiration in different sagittal planes (indicated by green vertical line). The pleura ascends up as one goes laterally. (A) Medially just lateral to the aorta; (B) Just medial to the midscapular line; (C) Lateral to the midscapular line

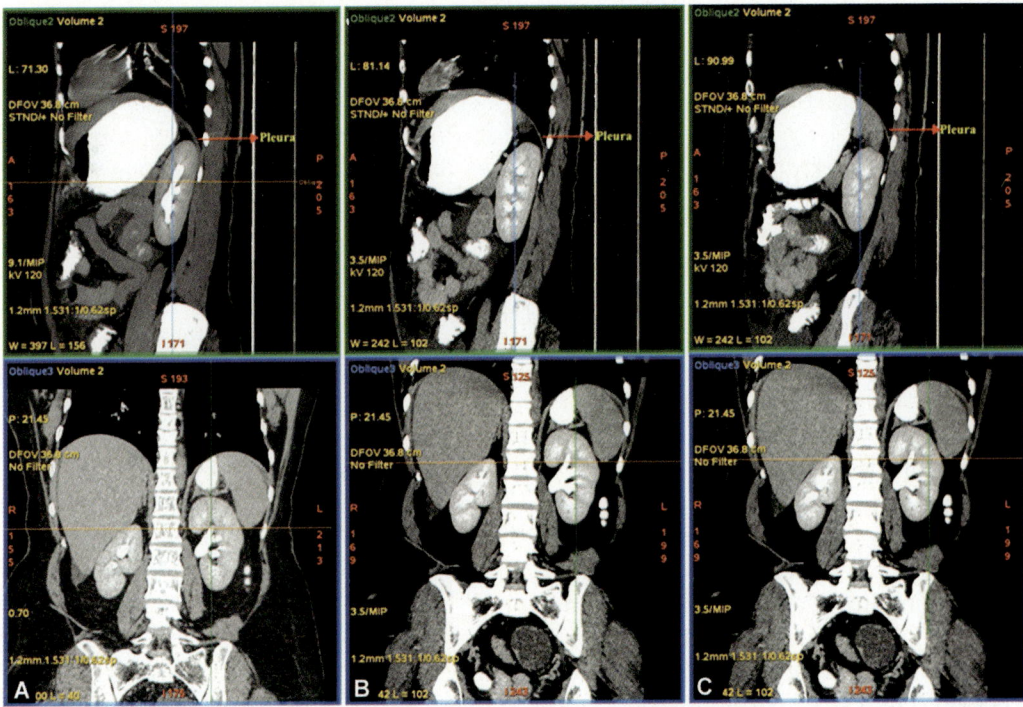

Fig. 1.10: Relationship of pleura with the upper pole of kidney during expiration in different sagittal planes (indicated by green vertical line). The pleura ascends up as one goes laterally. (A) Just medial to the midscapular line; (B) Midscapular line; (C) Lateral to the midscapular line

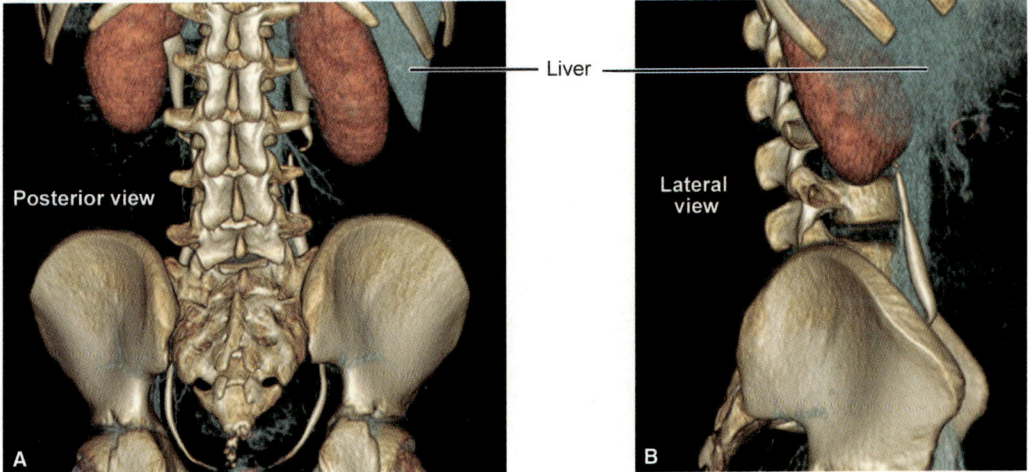

Fig. 1.11: Relationship of liver with kidney. (A) Posterior view: Posterior surface of kidney is free from the liver; (B) Lateral view: Liver covering the anterior surface of the kidney extends lateral to the kidney as well. A puncture too lateral or anterior can injure the liver

In one study of computed tomograms, the left colon was posterior in 16.1% of cases, and the right colon was posterior in 9% of cases at the level of the lower pole. At the midaspect of the kidney, the colon was posterior in 5.2% and 2.8%, respectively, and at the upper pole 1.1% and 0.4%, respectively. Hopper and colleagues, in a study of 500 CT scans of the abdomen,

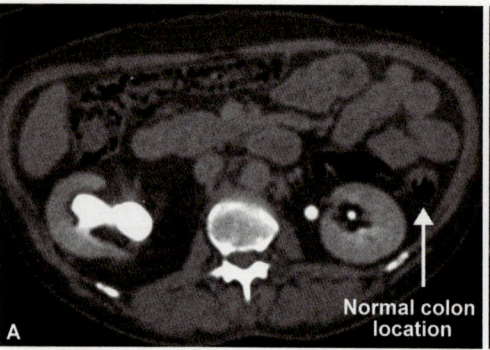 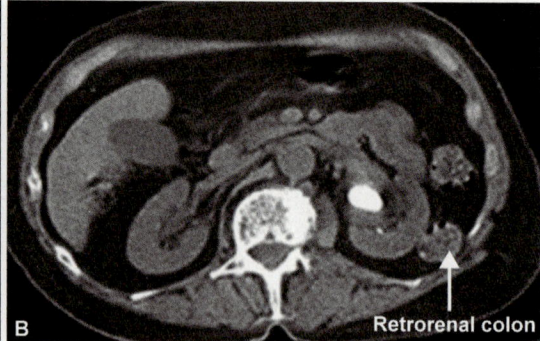

Fig. 1.12: Relationship of colon with kidney. (A) Normally the colon is anterior to the left kidney; (B) Retrorenal colon along the lower pole of left kidney

reported that the overall frequency of retrorenal colon in the supine patient was 1.9%.[8] When 90 patients were studied in the prone position, a retrorenal colon was found in 10%. A puncture placed too laterally may injure the colon. The position of the colon is usually anterior or anterolateral to the lateral renal border (Fig. 1.12). Therefore, risk of colon injury usually exists only with a very lateral (lateral to the posterior axillary line) puncture.

Additional visceral relations to the kidney include the adrenal glands (medial to the upper pole of both kidneys), the duodenum and gallbladder (anterior and medial to the right kidney), and the tail of the pancreas (anterior and medial to the left kidney). These structures can be injured with a misdirected or excessively deep puncture.

References

1. J Stuart Wolf. Percutaneous Approaches to the Upper Urinary Tract Collecting System. Campbell-Walsh Urology 11th edition.

2. Sampaio FJB. Surgical Anatomy of the Kidney in the Prone, Oblique, and Supine Positions. Smith's Textbook of Endourology, Third Edition:63–94.

3. Sampaio FJB, Mandarim-de-Lacerda CA. 3-Dimensional and radiological pelviocaliceal anatomy for endourology. J Urol. 1988;140:1352–1355.

4. Sampaio, F.J.B. Renal anatomy: Endourologic considerations. Urol Clin North Am, 2000;27:585–607.

5. Miller J, Durack JC, Sorensen MD, Wang JH, Stoller ML. Renal calyceal anatomy characterization with 3-dimensional in vivo computerized tomography imaging. J Urol. 2013;189:562–567.

6. Eisner BH, Cloyd J, Stoller ML. Lower-pole fluoroscopy-guided percutaneous renal access: which calix is posterior? J Endourol. 2009;23: 1621–1625.

7. Stening SG, Bourne S. Supracostal percutaneous nephrolithotomy for upper pole caliceal calculi. J Endourol. 1998;12;359–362.

8. Hopper KD, Sherman JL, Luethke JM, Ghaed N. The retrorenal colon in the supine and prone patient. Radiology. 1987;162:443–446.

Rajesh Kukreja

2 | Puncture of the Renal Pelvicalyceal System

HOW SHOULD AN IDEAL PUNCTURE BE?

An ideal puncture would fulfill all of the following criteria (Fig. 2.1):

1. The path should be a straight line from the skin passing through the cup of the calyx and the infundibulum to the pelvis.
2. It should traverse the minimum renal parenchyma.
3. It should give access to the maximum stone burden and the ureteropelvic junction when necessary.
4. There should be nil or minimal angulation or torque on the renal parenchyma and the infundibula.
5. Access should be from the cup or fornix of the posterior calyx. Such a puncture would traverse or traumatize the least and the smallest renal vessels. Puncture through the infundibulum of a calyx is associated with a significant risk of significant bleeding from interlobar vessels.
6. Puncture through the infundibulum of the upper, middle and lower poles was associated with vascular injury in 67.6%, 38.4% and 68.2% of kidneys, respectively. Puncture through the fornix proved to be much safer and it was associated with a venous injury rate of less than 8% and no arterial lesions. Direct puncture into the renal pelvis injured large retropelvic vessels in a third of cases and is also associated with potential prolonged urinary leakage and easy tube dislodgment.[1, 2]

The Ideal Initial Puncture Needle

The axial force of a needle during insertion in soft tissue is the summation of different forces distributed along the needle shaft such as

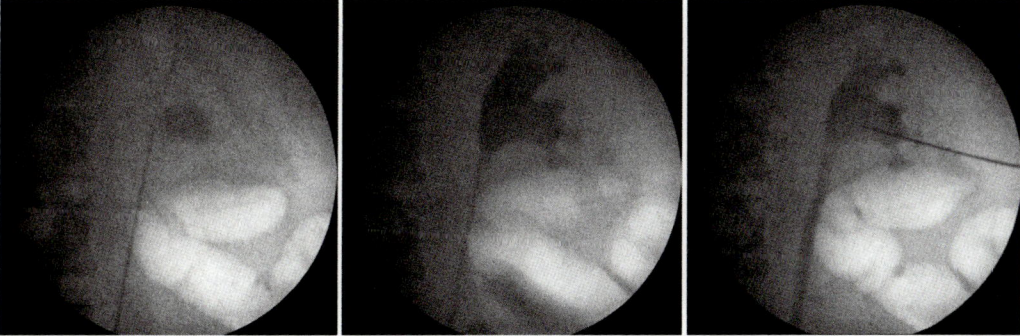

Fig. 2.1: An ideal puncture: The shortest distance from the skin to the cup of calyx in line with the infundibulum and renal pelvis and providing access to the maximum stone burden

stiffness force, frictional force and cutting force. Needle deflection and tissue deformation are major problems for accurate needle insertion.

- A diamond tip needle and not a bevel-tip needle should be used for the initial puncture. A diamond tip needle has symmetrical tip which exerts equal force in all directions on the tissue. Hence, the tissue is cut in the moving direction of the needle tip. A bevel-tip needle exerts forces asymmetrically, so cutting of the tissue occurs at an offset angle depending on the bevel angle, needle flexibility and tissue properties[3] (Fig. 2.2).
- The size of the needle used for puncture is a matter of debate. The options are a 21-gauge needle (which allows a 0.018 inch guidewire) or an 18 gauge needle (which allows a 0.035 inch guidewire). The 18 gauge needle is stiffer but more traumatic. The 21 gauge needle is less traumatic but less stiff and hence cannot maintain the trajectory adequately. Also, the 0.018 inch guidewire that passes through the 21 gauge needle must be exchanged for a standard 0.035 inch guide wire for subsequent tract dilatation. This requires an extra step, which adds to the complexity of the

procedure and increases the risk of loss of access. Weighing the pros and cons of both, it would be rational to use the 21 gauge needle when the surgeon is less experienced or if minimizing trauma is the need of the moment. The 18 gauge needle should be used by an experienced surgeon who is confident of attaining access with minimum attempts.[4]

- The safest initial 0.035 inch guidewire to use for upper urinary tract percutaneous access is a PTFE-coated J-wire. The "J" tip makes the guidewire unlikely to perforate out of the collecting system. This guidewire may not easily pass down the ureter, however. A floppy-tip PTFE-coated guidewire or a hydrophilic guidewire with a straight or angled tip passes down the ureter much easily.

Choosing the Correct Entry Calyx

- The calyx of entry should be selected based on the distribution of the stone to be treated. It should give access to the maximum stone burden and the ureteropelvic junction when necessary. The remaining stones if any can be addressed with a second (and rarely a third or more) access or with flexible instrumentation through the initial access site.
- An upper pole calyx is generally the most versatile site to enter the upper urinary tract collecting system. The renal pelvis, lower pole calyces, and ureter usually can be entered with a rigid nephroscope from a well-placed upper pole access. Percutaneous access into the upper pole is simplified by the more dense attachments of Gerota's fascia, reducing mobility, and the shorter distance from the skin compared to into the lower pole. Access to the middle calyces will usually require a separate access or use of flexible instrumentation.
- Middle calyceal entry offers adequate access to the pelvis, ureteropelvic junction and upper ureter.

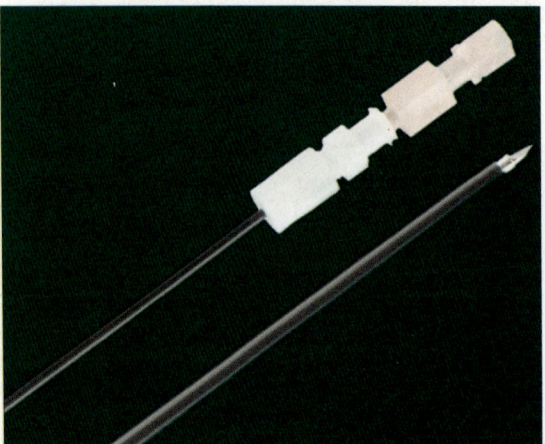
Fig. 2.2: Echotip diamond tip 18G needle (Cook Medical): The Echotip helps visualization during ultrasound-guided puncture

- Puncture of the lower pole may be slightly more difficult as the freely mobile lower pole moves away from the needle and dilators. Also, the lower pole tracts tend to be longer and more oblique, making stone removal from upper calyces with rigid instruments may be more difficult than the converse. Due to the posterior tilt of the upper pole of the kidney, the lower pole does not offer assured access to the upper pole.

Upper Calyceal Access: Subcostal or Supracostal

The upper portions of both the kidneys are located anterior to the posterior portion of the 11th and 12th ribs. A review of 90 normal supine intravenous urograms during full expiration noted that 85% of upper renal calyces are located above the 12th rib.[5] In the prone position, further cephalad movement of the kidney occurs in 80% of patients.[6]

Subcostal access is the safest route to the kidney because pleural injuries are rare with entry below the 12th rib. Nonetheless, if entry directly above the 12th rib (11th intercostal space) provides the best access to the optimal calyx, then the benefit generally exceeds the risk.

Entry above the 11th rib, however, has a greater potential for pleural and even lung injury, so when the best access calls for a direct puncture above the 11th rib, additional maneuvers could be considered to displace the kidney inferiorly. These include cephalad tilt of a subcostal access sheath placed into a lower calyx and attaining access during full inspiration. Smith et al[7] described the renal displacement technique wherein initial placement of a sheath or dilator is performed via a lower or midcalyx in order to allow for torque of the kidney downward. This can be held by an assistant while upper calyx puncture is performed via a subcostal route. This technique however mandates an unnecessary second tract. Another alternative is to angle the upper calyceal access tract cephalad from a subcostal skin entry site.

This approach provides limited access to the rest of the kidney and traverses more of the renal parenchyma obliquely with increased chances of bleeding.[8] All of these alternatives can result in severe angulation and torque on the renal infundibula with damage to the infundibular vessels.

Stening and Bourne have discussed in depth the anatomic considerations in the supracostal approach for renal surgery.[9] The lower limit of the parietal pleura crosses the 12th rib obliquely at its midpoint such that the lateral half of the rib is uncovered by the pleura. In the midscapular line, the visceral pleura is in relation to the 10th rib, while the parietal pleura is at the level of the 12th rib (Fig. 2.3). The parietal and visceral pleura ascend cranially and laterally on the ribs, and further rise in deep expiration. Thus, a puncture made lateral to the midscapular line, below the 10th rib, in deep expiration would almost always prevent damage to the visceral pleura (Fig. 2.4A).

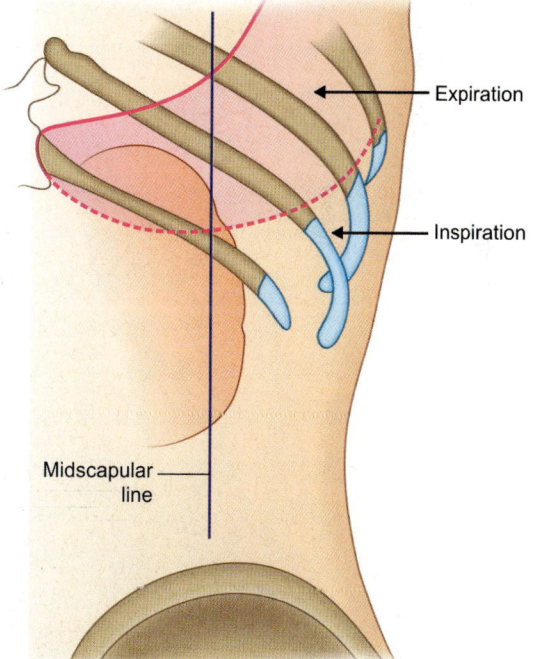

Fig. 2.3: Parietal pleura during phases of respiration: Diagrammatic representation (Stening and Bourne)

Based on the study by Stening and Bourne, important guidelines to reduce thoracic complications would be:

- All intercostal punctures should be done while the lung is deflated during expiration to decrease the risk of pulmonary injury.
- Supracostal access should be performed lateral to the midscapular line to minimize injury to the pleura[9–11] and in line with the calyx of entry, infundibulum and pelvis (Fig. 2.4B).
- The needle should be advanced along the upper margin of the rib during the expiratory phase. Needle passage along the inferior margin of the rib risks injury to the intercostal neurovascular bundle, which can result in significant bleeding.
- The supracostal skin puncture should be done over the lateral portion of the rib,

and the puncture should be made during steady, quiet breathing or breath holding in expiration. However, once the needle has passed the diaphragm, the calyceal entry can be made during full inspiration when the kidney descends caudally.[12]

- Access above the 10th rib is associated with a high incidence of pleural violation and lung injury and should be avoided unless absolutely necessary. Thoracoscopic guided access superior to the 10th rib can be performed to reduce the risk of lung injury.[13]

A multicenter retrospective study of patients undergoing percutaneous nephrolithotomy via upper pole access showed that patients with an intercostal approach experienced greater stone-free rates, fewer complications, and reduced operating times compared to patients with a subcostal approach.[14]

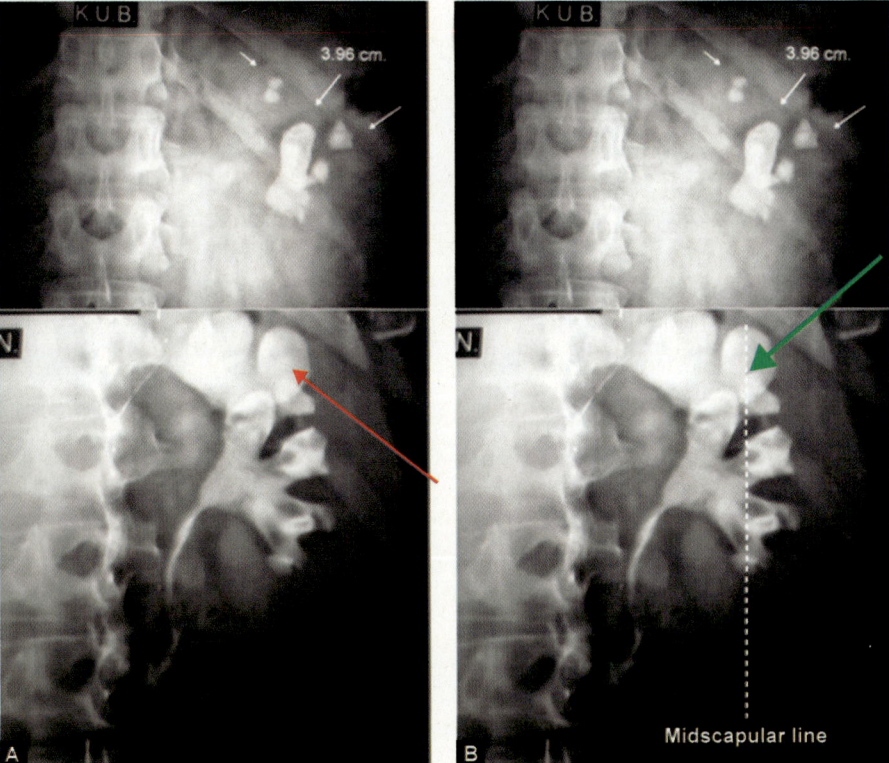

Fig. 2.4A and B: Upper calyceal puncture. (A) Incorrect angulated subcostal puncture; (B) Correct supracostal puncture with entry from lateral to the midscapular line

Risk of Visceral Injury

In the absence of splenomegaly or hepatomegaly injury to the liver and spleen is extremely rare when the access puncture site is below the 12th rib. However, supracostal access can be associated with an increased risk of injury to the liver and spleen, particularly if puncture is performed during the inspiratory phase of respiration rather than the expiratory phase or the puncture is above the 11th rib.[15, 16] To decrease the risk of liver or spleen injury, the skin puncture site should be located as far medial as possible.

Placement of Ureteric Catheter

A retrograde ureteric catheter delineates the ureteral anatomy, as well as the exact stone location, degree of hydronephrosis, and the image of the selected calyx in order to plan the approach to the collecting system.

Advantages of a retrograde ureteric catheter:

- Opacification of pelvicalyceal system.
- Prevents fragment migration down the ureter.
- Retrograde saline flushing during puncture, tract dilatation, and flushing out of fragments.
- Retrograde guidewires can be passed up if required.
- Injection of methylene blue for identification of the pelvic-ureteric junction (PUJ) or opening of calyceal diverticulum in difficult cases.

The rigid cystoscope is used to place a 0.038 inch Teflon-coated guidewire into the upper collecting system. When a tortuous area blocks the progress of the guidewire, a wire with a hydrophilic coating must be used. This wire is composed of an alloy core, a polyurethane jacket, and a thin hydrophilic polymer as the outer most layer. When in contact with fluid, the polymer binds water to create a lubricious coating with greatly diminished friction, avoiding excessive edema and creation of a false passage.[17] When the guidewire is in position, the 6F catheter is advanced over it

to the renal pelvis, and the endoscope is removed. A 16 F Foley catheter is inserted and attached to a drainage bag at the same time. Both the catheters are tied with 2–0 silk to secure them in place. It is helpful to connect an empty syringe to the Luer Lock adapter at the end of the ureteral catheter to prevent urine leakage.

Fluoroscopic Guided Access

There are two primary methods used to gain fluoroscopy-guided percutaneous renal access: The "bull's eye" technique and triangulation technique. Both the techniques need a target, most commonly generated by opacification of the collecting system with iodinated contrast that is administered retrograde via a ureteral catheter. A calyceal entry point is selected to avoid the larger vascular structures that are found at the level of the infundibulum.

Identifying the Posterior Calyx on Fluoroscopy

- Preoperative assessment with CT urogram or an IVU helps in identifying the posterior calyces.
- With the patient in prone position, diluted contrast when instilled will fill the dependent anterior calyces first. Thus, the posterior calyces will be filled later and would appear less dense. Injection of 5 to 10 ml of air via the ureteric catheter also helps to identify the posterior calyces as air will preferentially enter these calyces when the patient is prone.
- The movement of the C-arm can help to identify the posterior calyx. In the prone position, the posterior calyces move in the opposite direction to the image intensifier on the C-arm. If the C-arm is rotated toward the surgeon, then the posterior calyces move away and shorten. Vice versa, if the C-arm is rotated away from the surgeon, then the posterior calyces appear elongated. Thus, by moving the C-arm, way from the surgeon one can identify the

laterally placed calyces as posterior and by moving the C-arm toward the surgeon the posterior calyces appear more medially placed and appear end on.

Techniques[4, 17-20]

Bulls eye technique: With the C-arm in the 30° position, an 18 G diamond tip access needle is positioned, so that the targeted calyx, needle tip, and needle hub are in line with the image intensifier, giving a bulls eye effect on the monitor. In effect, the surgeon lookings down the needle into the targeted calyx. The needle is advanced to 1–2 cm increments using a hemostat to minimize radiation exposure to the surgeon. Continuous fluoroscopic monitoring is performed to ensure that the needle maintains its proper trajectory. Needle depth is ascertained by rotating the C-arm to a vertical orientation. If the needle is aligned with the calyx in this view, the urologist should be able to aspirate urine from the collecting system, confirming proper positioning.

The triangulation technique is based on simple geometric principles and is guided by biplanar fluoroscopy; one plane is anteroposterior (0°) to the line of puncture and the other is oblique (30°). The C-arm can be tilted oblique in any of the four directions:

- Toward or away from the surgeon at right angles to the operating table or
- Toward head end (cephalic) or foot end (caudal) of the patient parallel to the operating table.
- The anteroposterior view may be considered to be in a plane parallel to the axis of puncture and is used to monitor mediolateral (left-right) adjustments.
- The oblique view gives information regarding depth to the site of puncture and is used to monitor needle adjustments in the superficial/deep (posterior/anterior) orientation.
- When making adjustments in the mediolateral axis, care should be taken not to inadvertently move the needle in the cephalad caudad (superficial-deep) axis, and vice versa.
- It may be helpful for the surgeon to rest their arm on the patient during the access part of the procedure, as this minimizes unintended drifting of the needle away

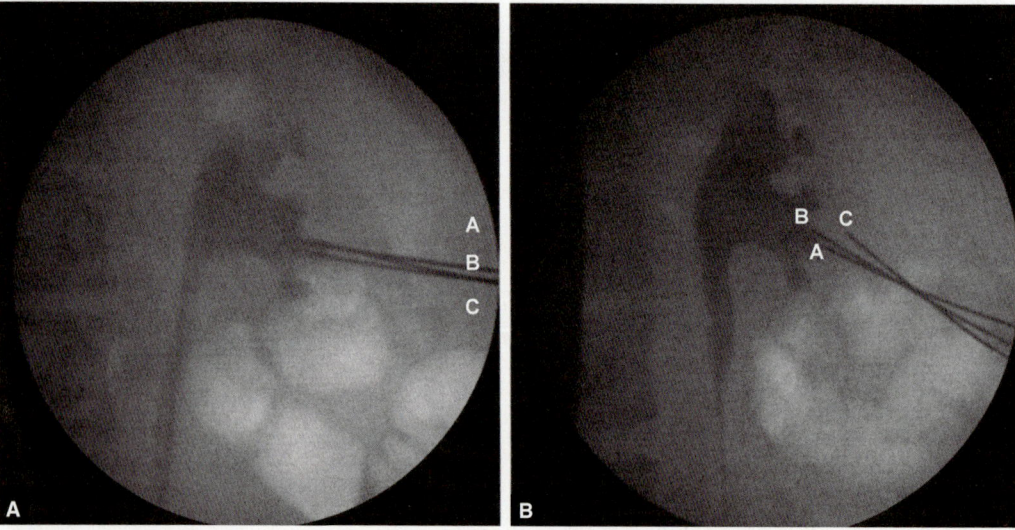

Fig. 2.5: (A) C-arm in 0°. All the 3 needles A, B, and C appear to be in the calyx. (C-arm in 30°); (B) Needle A is in the same calyx, needle B is posterior or superficial to the calyx (medial or towards the spine) and needle C is anterior or deep to the calyx (lateral or away from the spine)

from the targeted axis and also provides additional needle stabilization. Once the needle is aligned with the targeted calyx in both the mediolateral and cephalo-caudal (superficial-deep) orientations, it is advanced with continuous fluoroscopy.

- The needle should be advanced in the oblique view, which will allow for the assessment of the depth of the needle's penetration.
- It is helpful for the anesthesiologist to hold the patient's respirations while the needle is being advanced, to avoid having to "hit a moving target", as well as to minimize the risk of an inadvertent transthoracic puncture.
- After advancing the needle several centimeters in the oblique view, the anteroposterior view should be examined to confirm that the mediolateral trajectory of the needle is still properly aligned to the target. If necessary, the needle trajectory can be readjusted to maintain proper targeting.
- It is imperative that to minimize trauma to the renal parenchyma, the adjustment of the needle plane should be done when the needle is outside the renal capsule and not when the needle is in the parenchyma. Manipulating the needle after entering the renal parenchyma may displace and lacerate the kidney and alter the position of the targeted calyx. Again, it is critical not to alter the access needle's orientation in one plane while making adjustments in the other plane, particularly when advancing the needle.
- A slight jiggle of the needle causing indentation of the desired calyx is a further sign that the trajectory of the needle is correct.

Comparing the Two Techniques

- With the "eye-of-the-needle" technique, the proper cephalocaudal (superficial-deep) and mediolateral axes of the needle are verified and maintained on a single fluoroscopic view, and the confirmatory view is necessary only to assure the depth of the needle tip. For the "triangulation" technique, one fluoroscopic view is used to assess the mediolateral axis and another is used to assess the depth or cephalocaudal (superficial-deep) axis.[18]
- In the triangulation technique, the puncture is along the stone axis, i.e. in alignment with the infundibulum. This decreases the need for excessive torque on the renal paren-chyma by the rigid instruments, which may cause renal trauma and bleeding. Tepeler et al[21] did a comparison of the bull's eye and the triangulation technique and found no difference between the two as regards operation time, fluoroscopy screening time, duration of hospitalization and blood transfusion rate. They found a slightly greater drop in hematocrit and complication rate in the group undergoing access by the bull's eye technique as compared to the triangulation technique. However, the difference was not statistically different.
- The advantage of the triangulation technique over the "eye-of-the-needle" technique is that the needle cannot be passed too deeply because the depth of advancement is monitored continuously. Also, the triangu-lation technique alone fulfills the five criteria of a successful puncture.
- The disadvantage of the triangulation technique is that maintaining both the mediolateral and cephalocaudal (superfi-cial-deep) planes are difficult because both are not being monitored at the same time as in the "eye-of-the-needle" technique. Multiple attempts with excessive use of fluoroscopy may occur especially with a beginner. Usually, during the learning curve the problem comes in the assessment of superficial-deep planes with the C-arm in the oblique position. Whether the needle is superficial-deep to the calyx, has to be

ascertained by the surgeon and adjustments made accordingly. The easiest way to determine this would be to place another needle on the skin surface over the target calyx or correlate with the spine. If the calyx is between the two needles or between the spine and the puncture needle, then the puncture needle is deep and should be adjusted superficially. If the target calyx is below the two needles or below the puncture needle and the spine, then the puncture needle is superficial and should be adjusted toward the depth.

Hybrid Technique[19]

- The three most important things needed to achieve a successful percutaneous renal puncture are the site of skin entry, the angle of entry and the depth at which the puncture is achieved.
- Determining the correct point of skin puncture is important in the triangulation technique because a skin puncture that is too medial or lateral to the desired optimum point of entry would result in a tract of variable length and angle of entry in the calyx. This would interfere with proper access and would cause excessive torque on the parenchyma during maneuvering of the rigid nephroscope in the pelvicalyceal system. To avoid injury to the colon, the puncture should be medial to the posterior axillary line but not too medial as it would traverse the paraspinal muscle causing increased postoperative pain and would probably be directly on the renal pelvis without traversing the renal parenchyma. The puncture that is too close to the rib may injure the intercostal nerve and vessels and hence is to be avoided.
- Sharma described the technique of determining the site of skin puncture, which amalgamates the advantages of both the bull's eye and triangulation technique and hence is called the hybrid technique. With the C-arm at 0°, the site of skin

corresponding to the target calyx is marked as point A. The C-arm is then rotated 30° towards the surgeon. The point on the skin corresponding to the target calyx and forming a bull's eye with the needle is marked as point B. In the bull's eye technique we take a puncture at the point B. However, in the triangulation technique, the puncture is along the stone axis in alignment with the infundibulum. If we take the target calyx as the center of a sphere, then we have an imaginary circle on the skin where the point A is the center of the circle. The distance from point A to B will be the radius of the circle. The radius remains the same irrespective of the direction in which it is measured from the center of the circle. Thus, when we take a line along the stone axis where we intend to take a puncture—the site of skin puncture is marked using this principle. This means that the point B1 is marked on the skin such that the distance from point A to B1 is equal to the distance between A to B, i.e. the radius of a circle with the target calyx being its center. B1 is the site of entry on the skin.

- The angle of puncture: In the bull's eye technique, the angle at which the needle is seen as a dot is the angle at which the puncture is made. The hybrid technique utilizes this principle. With the needle at point B and the C-arm rotated 30° towards the surgeon and the needle forming the bull's eye; the angle that the needle makes with the skin surface is measured using a protractor. One needs to take care that the protractor is held parallel to the operating table. Using the principle of sphere and circle; if we are hitting the calyx by using the triangulation technique from the point B1—the angle of puncture would be the same with probably variations of 1–2° due to the not so perfectly flat contours of the body surface.
- The third component of the hybrid technique is to determine the depth of

puncture. What we have till now is an imaginary triangle where we know: (1) One side—the distance between point A to B which is marked on the skin; (2) One angle, which is 90° with the C-arm at 0°; and (3) Another angle, which is measured using the protractor at the point B. With this information; by using the universal triangle solver application from Google play store we can determine the depth. In this application, if we put the two angles and one side then, by the law of sines, it calculates the other two sides and the angle. For example, if the distance AB is 4 cm and the angle calculated by the protractor is 65° and with the other angle always being 90° by universal triangle solver—the depth will be 9.5 cm.

Confirmation of an Ideal Posterior Calyceal Puncture

- If air has been instilled during opacification of the pelvicalyceal system, sudden release of air followed by a free flow of clear saline instilled through the ureteric catheter.
- When the glide wire is passed maintaining the angle of the needle, it enters the pelvis easily. No manipulation is needed. On the contrary if the anterior calyx has been punctured than the glide wire will be coiled in the calyx, will not enter the pelvis easily or will do so only after much manipulation.
- If at the point of withdrawing the trocar of the needle spontaneous output of urine has not been observed, it is advisable gently to try to introduce a hydrophilic guidewire, observing the advancement of the guidewire under fluoroscopy. Typically, it moves into the cavity of the calyx and progresses towards the renal pelvis.
- If no urine exits from the 18G needle and even a hydrophilic guidewire cannot be negotiated into the pelvicalyceal system, the needle is unlikely to be correctly placed. It is not advisable to inject contrast through the needle, since contrast can extravasate,

creating a lake of radio-opaque material and making subsequent visualization of the pelvicalyceal system difficult.

- Complex situations: In situations where the volume of the stone occupies the entire volume of the calyx selected to be punctured, the needle is advanced until there is the tactile sensation of the needle tip touching the hard surface of the stone. In this situation the tip of the trocar of the needle is in contact with the stone but the cannula of the needle is at a distance of 1–2 mm from the surface of the stone. It is advisable to move the cannula on the trocar towards the stone until contact with the surface of the stone is felt. Then the trocar needle is removed and the hydrophilic guidewire is gently inserted into the narrow space between the urothelium of the calyx and the surface of the stone. Sometimes this allows the advancement of the guidewire to the renal pelvis, but in other situations it is only possible to locate the guidewire in the punctured calyx.

Multiple Tracts

In the treatment of complex renal lithiasis with branches in multiple calyces, it is sometimes necessary to make multiple punctures through different calyces. Proper assessment of the pelvicalyceal system and planning of the tracts is a must. Multiple punctures when deemed probable should all be made initially. If the planned multiple punctures are made at the beginning of surgery, the injection of contrast through the initially placed ureteral catheter facilitates visualization of all calyces and the most suitable for punctures can be chosen in accordance with the silhouette of the stone. The injection of contrast distends the upper urinary tract and this facilitates insertion of the needles into the calyces. In contrast, if secondary punctures are made after debulking of the stone through the initial primary tract, the calyceal distension of the cavities may be hampered by the leaking of contrast and saline that is injected from the ureteral catheter through the Amplatz sheath.

If calculi are located in calyces that are in parallel with or adjacent to the calyx of initial puncture, a Y puncture technique, in which the secondary puncture angles off of the initial nephrostomy tract, may be considered.[18] After the calyx of initial puncture is cleared of stone the working sheath is retracted outside of the renal capsule and angled towards the second targeted calyx. The second puncture is made through the working sheath. One of the attractions of the Y puncture is that the second puncture is created through the same skin incision as the first puncture, minimizing the cosmetic effects of PNL. We do not advocate this technique as the second tract would become oblique with higher risk of bleeding and vascular injury. It is better to have two separate skin entry points and reduce the amount of parenchyma traversed.

ULTRASOUND-GUIDED ACCESS

Percutaneous renal access can be achieved either with ultrasound or fluoroscopy guidance. The method of choice depends on training and personal preference. The side effects of extensive radiation during therapeutic procedures are well-known, which is the main drawback of fluoroscopy.

Ultrasound has several strengths as an interventional tool.[22]

- It is readily available, relatively in expensive, and portable.
- It has no radiation hazards.
- It provides guidance for access in multiple, transverse, longitudinal, and oblique planes.
- It offers real time monitoring of the needle tip, which guides proper placement of the needle and avoidance of important viscera.
- An added advantage is that it can be used in conjunction with Doppler to avoid important vascular structures lying along the needle path.

- Percutaneous ultrasound-guided access is the simplest and most direct technique to drain a hydronephrotic collecting system in difficult clinical conditions as in placing a temporary urinary diversion due to an obstructing stone with infection, pyonephrosis or renal failure. It has also been used successfully to relieve upper tract obstruction secondary to malignancy. Ultrasound-guided nephrostomy puncture is preferred for patients in whom retrograde ureteral access is unsuccessful. It is also a method of choice in pregnancy when there is a need for deobstruction.

In a few comparative studies,[23–27] ultrasound-guided access has been associated with reduced radiation exposure time, reduced number of attempts to puncture and reduced blood loss as compared to fluoroscopy-guided access. Urologists trained in percutaneous access may be able to provide improved stone-free rates during percutaneous nephrolithotomy (PCNL) while minimizing access related complications.

Instrumentation

Convex probes produce rectangular scans and are most commonly used for gaining percutaneous renal access. Sector probes can be useful when performing nephrostomies in the pediatric age group. The ideal transducer for renal access is a convex transducer of 3.5 MHz, focused at 7–9 cm. If children or thin patients are to be scanned, then a 5-MHz smaller transducer with a focus at 5–7 cm is required. Alternatively, a sector probe can be used in this situation. The monitor used for intervention should ideally be equipped with an electronic dotted line which shows the needle path.

The rigidity of the 18 G needle compared to the 21 G needle is advantageous for accurately directing the needle tip as it is advanced through the fascial planes. The 18 G needle tip is also readily identifiable with real-time ultrasonography guidance. Although routine needles can be used for this purpose, the echo tip needle (Cook Medical Inc., Bloomington, IN, USA) is helpful in achieving ultrasound-guided access; the needle tip is scored and this increases the reflectivity and visualization on ultrasound. Clear visibility of the needle is "key" to the success of ultrasound-guided needle access (Fig. 2.6). The most common reason for non-visualization of the needle tip is nonalignment of the needle tip and transducer. This can be achieved by proper alignment using a puncture guide.

Technique (Fig. 2.6)

Ultrasound scanning commences posteriorly and proceeds until the posterior axillary line. If scanned in this way, the first calyx to be seen will be the posterior calyx. The site of needle entry is marked and the puncture performed with an 18 G echo tip (Cook Medical Incorporated) needle. The key point at this crucial step is that there should be minimal respiratory and ultrasound probe movement. In order to ensure an accurate puncture, the needle tip should be seen along the electronic dotted line throughout its course. The position of the needle in the desired calyx is confirmed with return of clear fluid.

Ultrasound-guided access satisfies all the attributes of a perfect renal access, i.e. shortest possible tract traversing the skin, cortex of the kidney, and cup of the desired calyx of puncture in a straight line and in alignment with the infundibulum and renal pelvis.

Ultrasound Punctures in Ectopic Kidneys and Transplanted Kidneys

A supine oblique position with a bolster under the ipsilateral hemipelvis is used. A mechanical bowel preparation with a low enema is used in all the cases. This helps in identification of gas in the sigmoid colon, which helps identify the bowel and prevents possible injury. Pressure on the ultrasound probe helps to displace the intervening bowel loops between the puncture line and targeted calyx. Similarly, contralateral pressure applied by the assistant helps displace the kidney close to the abdominal wall. All these maneuvers improve the chances of achieving a straight, short, and direct tract to the desired calyx. PCNL is feasible in transplanted kidneys with the help of ultrasound-guided access and this decreases the amount of radiation and intravenous contrast required. With the patient in a left-sided oblique position with a bolster under the ipsilateral hip, the bowel is displaced and a puncture into the superior calyx provides easy access to the ureteropelvic junction and stone in the pelvis.

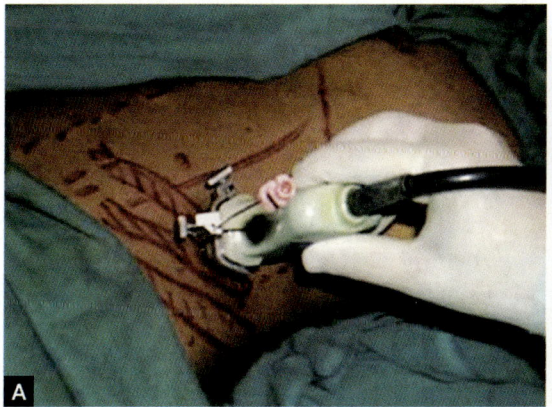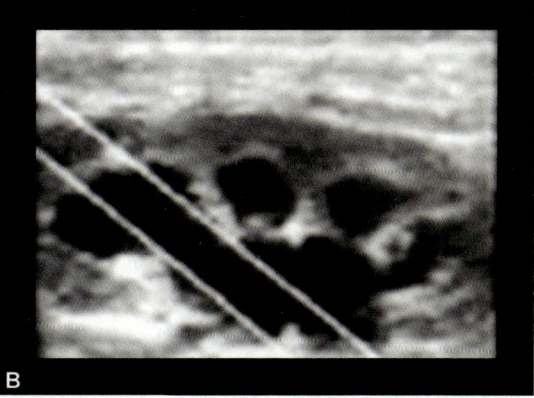

Fig. 2.6A and B: (A) The puncture guide helps in directing the needle in the desired plane and depth; (B) The ultrasound probe should be aligned in such a way that the tract provides the shortest access from the skin through the cup of the calyx, infundibulum, and finally into the pelvis

The addition of Doppler to ultrasound imaging (which facilitates visualization of blood vessels) may be associated with less blood loss and/or lower transfusion rate than ultrasound alone.[28]

BLIND ACCESS

The upper urinary tract collecting system can also be accessed "blindly," without any imaging guidance.[29] The only situation in which this should be considered is when sonography is not available and there is complete ureteral obstruction (precluding retrograde instillation of contrast material or opacification of the collecting system with intravenous contrast). The lumbar notch, also known as the superior lumbar triangle or Grynfeltt lumbar triangle, has been reported as a reliable landmark for blind percutaneous renal access. The lumbar notch is an area of muscular insufficiency through which hernias can occur. It is located posteriorly below the 12th rib. The superior border is the 12th rib and the latissimus dorsi muscle, the lateral border is the transversus abdominis and external oblique muscles, the medial border is the quadratus lumborum and sacrospinalis muscles, and the inferior border is the internal oblique muscle. Insert a needle 3 to 4 cm deep into the notch at a 30° cephalad angle to enter the collecting system. Another blind approach to the collecting system is to insert a needle directly perpendicular to the body surface 1 to 1.5 cm lateral to the L1 vertebral body, which will lead directly to the renal pelvis if anatomy is normal. If fluoroscopy is available, then air and contrast material can be injected through a blindly placed needle to assess fluoroscopically its position and to guide another needle properly through a posterior calyx. In the only randomized clinical trial comparing "blind" access to image-guided access, entry into the collecting system was successful in 50% and 90% of cases, respectively.[30] Use of the technique is not recommended in most settings.

References

1. Sampaio FJB. Surgical Anatomy of the Kidney in the Prone, Oblique, and Supine Positions. Smith's Textbook of Endourology, Third Edition:63–94.

2. Sampaio FJB, Mandarim-de-Lacerda CA. 3-Dimensional and radiological pelviocaliceal anatomy for endourology. J Urol 1988;140:1352–55.

3. Abolhassani N, Patel R, Moallem M. Needle insertion into soft tissue: a survey. Med Eng Phys 2007;29:413–31.

4. Wolf JS. Percutaneous approaches to the upper urinary tract collecting system. Campbell-Walsh Urology. 10th ed. Philadelphia, PA: Saunders Elsevier; 2011.

5. Payne, S.R., Webb, W.R. Percutaneous Renal Surgery, 2nd edn. Edinburgh: Churchill Livingstone, 1988, pp. 5–6.

6. Preminger, G.M., Schulez, S., Clayman, R.V., et al. Cephaladrenal movement during percutaneous nephrostolithotomy. J Urol 1986;137:623–25.

7. Karlin, G.S., Smith, A.D. Approaches to the superior calyx: Renal displacement technique and review of options. J Urol 1989;142:774–77.

8. Ahmed R. El-Nahas, Ahmed A. Shokeir, et al. Post-percutaneous Nephrolithotomy Extensive Hemorrhage: A Study of Risk Factors. J Urol 2007; 177: 576.

9. Stening SG, Bourne S. Supracostal percutaneous nephrolithotomy for upper pole calyceal calculi. J Endourol 1998;12;359–62.

10. Yates J and Munver R. Diagnosis and Management of Thoracic Complications of Percutaneous Renal Surgery. Smith's Textbook of Endourology, third edition.

11. Maheshwari PN, Mane DA, Pathak AB. Management of pleural injury after percutaneous renal surgery. J Endourol 2009;23:1769–72.

12. El-Nahas, A.R., Shokeir, A.A., El-Kenawy, M.R., et al. Safety and efficacy of supracostal percutaneous nephrolithotomy in pediatric patients. J Urol 2008;180:676–680.

13. Finelli A, Honey RJDA. Thoracoscopy-assisted high intercostal percutaneous renal access. J Endourol 2001;15:581–85.

14. Lang E, Thomas R, Davis R, et al. Risks, advantages, and complications of intercostal vs subcostal approach for percutaneous nephrolithotripsy. Urology 2009;74:751–55.

15. Hopper KD and Yakes WF. The posterior intercostal approach for percutaneous renal procedures: risk of puncturing the lung, spleen, and liver as determined by CT. AJR Am J Roentgenol 1990; 154: 115.

16. Robert M, Maubon A, Roux JO, Rouanet JP, Navratil H. Direct percutaneous approach to the upper pole of the kidney: MRI anatomy with assessment of the visceral risk. J Endourol 1999; 13: 17.

17. Bernardo NO. Percutaneous Renal Access Under Fluoroscopic Control. Smith's Textbook of Endourology. 3rd ed.

18. Miller NL, Matlaga BR, Lingeman JE. Techniques for fluoroscopic percutaneous renal access. J Urol 2007;178:15–23.

19. Sharma G, Sharma A. Determining site of skin puncture for percutaneous renal access using fluoroscopy-guided triangulation technique. J Endourol 2009;23:193–95.

20. Steinberg PL, Semins MJ, Wason SE, Matlaga BR, Pais VM. Fluoroscopy-guided percutaneous renal access. J Endourol 2009;23:1627–31.

21. Tepeler A, Armagan A, Akman T, Polat EC, Ersöz C, Topakta R, Erdem MR, Onol SY. Impact of percutaneous renal access technique on outcomes of percutaneous nephrolithotomy. J Endourol 2012;26:828–33.

22. Desai MR, Ganpule AP. Percutaneous Renal Access Under Ultrasound Control. Smith's Textbook of Endourology. 3rd ed.

23. Basiri, A., Ziaee, A.M., Kianian, H.R., et al. Ultrasonographic versus fluoroscopic access for percutaneous nephrolithotomy:A randomized clinical trial. J Endourol 2008;22:281–84.

24. Zegel, H.G., Pollack, H.M., Banner, M.C., et al. Percutaneous nephrostomy: Comparison of sonographic and fluoroscopic guidance. AJR Am J Roentgenol 1981;137:925–27.

25. Kukreja, R., Desai, M., Patel, S., et al. Factors affecting blood loss during percutaneous nephrolithotomy: prospective study. J Endourol 2004;18:715–22.

26. Agarwal M, Agrawal MS, Jaiswal A, et al. Safety and efficacy of ultrasonography as an adjunct to fluoroscopy for renal access in percutaneous nephrolithotomy (PCNL). BJU Int. 2011;108:1346–49.

27. Watterson, J.D., Soon, S., Jana, K. Access related complications during percutaneous nephro-lithotomy: urology versus radiology at a single academic institution. J Urol 2006;176:142–45.

28. Tzeng B-C, Wang C-J, Huang S-W, et al. Doppler ultrasound-guided percutaneous nephrolithotomy: a prospective randomized study. Urology 2011; 78:535–39.

29. Chien GW, Bellman GC. Blind percutaneous renal access. J Urol 2002;16:93–96.

30. Basiri A, Mehrabi S, et al. Blind Puncture in comparison with fluoroscopic guidance in PCNL: a randomized controlled trial. Uro J 2007;4:79–83.

3 | Positional and Anesthetic Considerations

Rajesh Kukreja

Goodwin and colleagues (1955) described the prone position for percutaneous access to the upper urinary tract collecting system.[1] The majority of PCNLs are carried out in general anesthesia with the patient in the prone position, with prior retrograde placement of a ureteral catheter in supine lithotomy position.[2]

PRONE POSITIONING

The prone position has been the standard position for PCNL due to the various advantages it offers.

Advantages of Prone Position

1. Presenting a large surface area (the patient's back) that provides many choices of access sites especially for upper calyceal approach and a stable horizontal working surface.
2. Most direct one to the desirable posterior calyces and comes closest to approaching the kidney through the Brödel avascular line.
3. More distended collecting system because of the effects of gravity on the irrigating fluid.
4. Unrestricted range of movement for the nephroscope.

Prone positioning does have some disadvantages as well

1. It is associated with a decrease in cardiac index.
2. The anesthesiologist has poor access to the airway with the patient in the prone position.
3. Prone positioning might not be possible in patients with morbid obesity and/or spinal concavity.
4. It can be associated with neuromusculo-skeletal complications such as nerve compression or stretch injury, ocular or facial injury, and rhabdomyolysis.

Physiologic changes to anesthetized patients in the prone position

1. There is more uniform distribution of pulmonary blood flow, improving ventilation to perfusion matching and oxygenation.[3–5] Also, functional residual capacity increases (compared to the anesthetized supine position) in normal weight and less so in obese patients.[3–5] Care must be taken to position chest rolls so that abdominal contents and the chest wall can move freely, or mechanical obstruction to ventilation may occur, increasing peak airway pressures and inhibiting effective mechanical ventilation.
2. Direct pressure to the abdominal contents may also be injurious, causing decrease in visceral perfusion. Such mechanical

compression has been reported to cause ischemia.

3. Patient's mean arterial pressure (MAP) often decreases in the prone position. This has been thought to be due to decreases in cardiac index (CI) and stroke volume.[3–5] The prone position impedes venous return and/or impedes left ventricular outflow during systole as a result of increased intrathoracic pressure. In either case, the decrease in CI is usually well-tolerated in healthy individuals with good cardiac reserve, due to reflexive increases in systemic vascular resistance and MAP. However, in those with poor cardiovascular reserve, vasopressor support may be indicated to maintain perfusion pressure. Significant hemodynamic changes can be expected if patients have an increased body mass index (BMI), cardiac or respiratory co-morbidities, and/or are suboptimally positioned.

• Patient-related risk factors include decreased neck mobility, fixed cardiac outflow obstruction, pulmonary hypertension, chronic airflow obstruction, and morbid obesity with large abdominal pannus.

• Proper positioning with chest and lower abdominal bolsters ensures minimal effect on venous return, leaving the abdominal contents and thorax freely mobile. This protects the intra-abdominal contents from pressure and facilitates positive pressure ventilation by allowing full diaphragmatic excursion and full lung expansion (Fig. 3.1A). The 'Montreal' mattress (Fig. 3.1B), which can be easily mounted on any operating table, is a rectangular mattress with a central hollow which helps to prevent compression of the abdomen during respiration and avoids interference with the venous

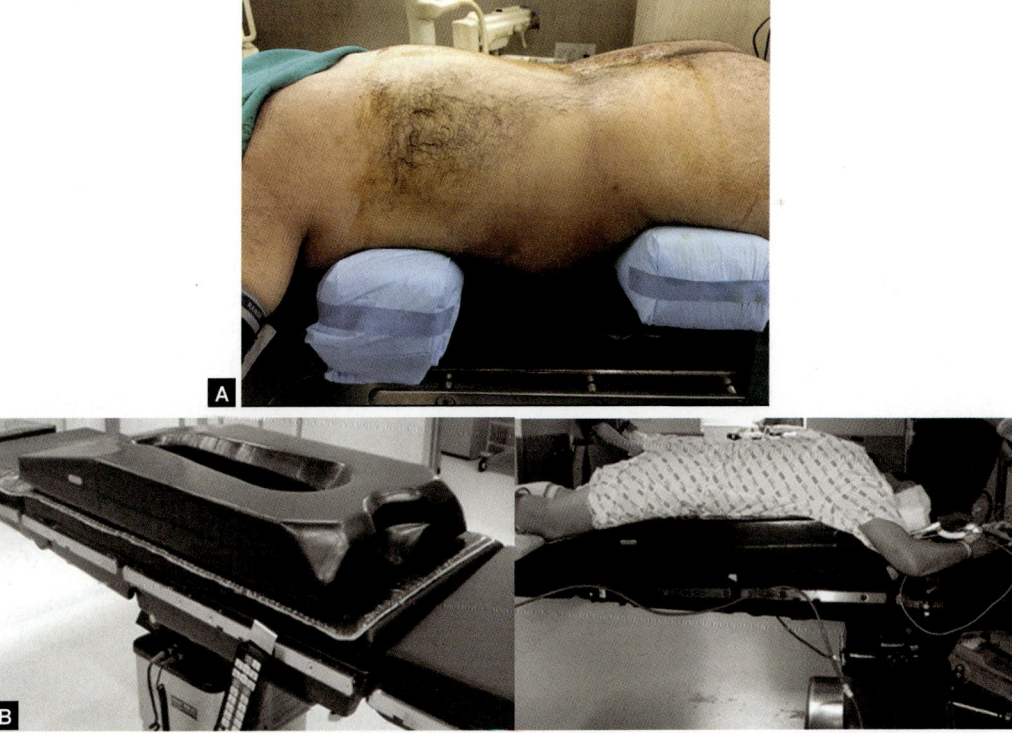

Fig. 3.1A and B: (A) Foam bolsters one below the lower chest and one below the pelvis; (B) Montreal mattress

return. It has a gutter at the head end to ensure mild flexion of the neck, assisting airway maintenance. Flexion at the hips is facilitated by slight slope towards the lower end.

Airway Maintenance

- Prone positioning requires that the patient's face be maintained free of pressure on prominences (eyes, nose, ears, cheekbones), with appropriate cushioning and support.
- The cervical spine must be maintained in a neutral position.
- The endotracheal tube must be taped securely at an appropriate depth and positioned free of kinks or pressure so that there is no obstruction within the airway during patient repositioning or during the procedure. A bite block should be placed between upper and lower molars (or gums if patient is edentulous) to prevent patient biting on the tongue, soft tissues, or endotracheal tube. The trachea must be positioned without pressure or risk of impeding a patent the patient airway.
- One useful commercial device that serves all these purposes is the ProneView® ProtectiveHelmet system (Dupaco, UK) (Fig. 3.2). This device is used for head and face positioning and incorporates a padded cradle, supported by short posts, with a mirror underneath to allow easy visualization of the patient's face and endotracheal tube.
- Prone position head gel beds are also available.
- Longer PCNL procedures may lead to significant dependent edema to inferiorly located anatomy. Upper airway edema and macroglossia can result from local compression (e.g. oral airways), venous or lymphatic obstruction (from neck rotation/hyperflexion), and tissue hypoperfusion due to systemic hypotension. In addition, edematous tissues bleed easily during attempts to re-establish the airway. Finally, coughing and laryngospasm can further compromise the upper airway. If there is concern regarding supraglottic airway edema, extubation should be delayed until the edema has resolved significantly. This may be evaluated by an endotracheal tube "leak check" to ensure sufficient ventilation exchange around the endotracheal tube with cuff deflated. In most patients, a brief period of head elevation during recovery is sufficient to remove the edema.[3]

Complications Related to Changing Position

Turning the patient prone is often accompanied by a temporary loss of patient monitoring, and can be associated with dislodgement of the endotracheal tube (ETT) and other intravenous or arterial catheters. Oxygen desaturation may occur during the subsequent unventilated period. Maintaining patients on 100% O_2 before position change can mitigate this problem by providing more oxygen reserves. Temporary disconnection of the breathing circuital interrupts the delivery of inhaled anesthetics and can increase the risk of patient awareness. In addition, physical injuries to the patient and staff may occur during positioning. It is important to provide adequate and specific training to all members of the OR team to reduce the risk of this occurring.[3, 4]

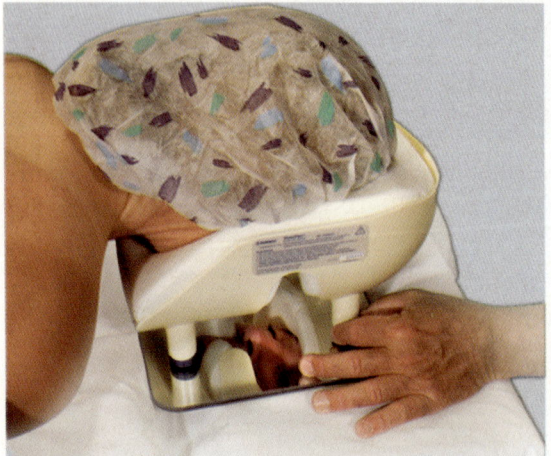

Fig. 3.2: ProneView® ProtectiveHelmet system (Dupaco, UK)

Variations of Prone Position

A. *Prone Flexed Position*[2, 6]

The patient is then placed in the prone position, and the table flexed 30 to 40° to open the space between the 12th rib and the posterior iliac crest.

Advantages

1. The working distance between the PSIC and the 12th rib is further increased.
2. The kidneys are displaced inferiorly in the retroperitoneum. This effect is most pronounced with the left kidney, which was lower than the right in 92.3% of cases. Because of this modification, a supra 11th rib access may be converted to a supra 12th rib or a supra 12th to an infracostal access.
3. The flank is significantly flattened, eliminating interference from the buttock during lower pole access.

B. *Prone Split Leg Position*

A split-leg modification can facilitate access to the external genitalia, for simultaneous antegrade and retrograde approaches.

SUPINE POSITION

Valdivia Uria and colleagues first reported the supine approach to percutaneous nephrolithotomy in 1987 and presented their review of 557 patients with percutaneous nephrolithotomy performed in this position.[7, 8] They reported few complications; there were no hydrothoraces or pneumothoraces, no colon injuries, and only a 0.5% rate of major hemorrhage.

Proposed advantages of the supine position include

1. The access sheath is angled towards horizontal (compared with vertical during percutaneous nephrolithotomy in the prone position), which reduces the pressure in the collecting system and facilitates stone fragments to wash out through the sheath.
2. Does not require repositioning after induction of anesthesia.
3. The urethra is more easily accessed than in the prone position.
4. Combined simultaneous antegrade and retrograde accesses are possible.
5. Safer position with regard to neuromusculoskeletal complications, and the anesthesia team may prefer this position.[10]
6. Because the percutaneous entry is more lateral than during a prone procedure, the instruments are closer to the surgeon, which results in less physical strain on the surgeon and the opportunity for the surgeon to sit during the procedure.

There are some disadvantages to the supine position for percutaneous renal surgery

1. It is not familiar to most urologists because the prone position is used in most training programs.
2. The reduced pressure in the collecting system results in a lower volume and thus less room for visualization and manipulation. Dependent nephrostomy drainage in this position also results in a collapsed system, often containing air bubbles that may interfere with visualization.
3. Stone fragments also collect in the dependent posterior calyces rather than the renal pelvis, as is the case when the patient is prone.
4. Upper pole calyceal access is more difficult in the supine compared with prone position.
5. The percutaneous tract length is longer than in the prone position.[11]
6. Restricted range of movements of the nephroscope due to clashing against the operating table and patient's hips. Some nephroscopes are short (<20 cm) and are not recommended, as they receive light and

water connections from opposite sides, which cause problems for the positioning of bag or the patient's hip, and obstructs the tilting movements of the endoscope.

7. With optimal placement of pads and bolsters, the prone position may provide better ventilation than the supine position.[5, 10]

POSITIONING[7-9]

Once anesthetized, the patient is pulled down the table and the legs placed in the lithotomy position. The ipsilateral hip is flexed with a flexed knee, and the contralateral leg is abducted and supported in an extended position. The beanbag is rolled under the hips and shoulders to tilt and support the torso at approximately 20 to 30°. The ipsilateral arm is supported with a flexed elbow over the chest with the contralateral arm tucked next to the torso with an extended elbow. This original position does not allow for easy concurrent retrograde instrumentation and also provides limited space for choosing an access.

Dr. Gaspar Ibarluzea, from Bilbao, Spain, modified this position with slight lateralization of the Valdivia decubitus position with extension of the ipsilateral leg and flexion of the contralateral lower limb. This decubitus position is called Valdivia-Galdakao decubitus position. This allows access to the entire urinary tract without the need for repositioning and allows simultaneous retrograde access.

Many supine positions have been developed, including the complete supine, Valdivia, Galdakao modified Valdivia, Barts modified (90° flank rotation offering wide surface area for access but makes the puncture more difficult due to end on calyces superimposed with the spine) and Barts flank-free modified supine (15° flank elevation with 5–10° C-arm rotation) positions; all aiming at improving flank exposure to allow for easy and multiple punctures. Supine PCNL positions are nearly similar; putting the patient in the supine position by elevating the flank up to 20° and thus causing the posterior calyx to project more laterally often becoming parallel (30°) to the fluoroscopy table. It is important that the edge of the bag and the patient's flank are alongside the surgical table edge, in order to facilitate the free movement of the nephroscope.

THE FLANK (LATERAL DECUBITUS) POSITION

This was first described by Kerbl[12] and colleagues and is less commonly used for percutaneous renal surgery. This position allows simultaneous access to the anterior and posterior aspects of the kidney and appears to be particularly useful for morbidly obese patients or those with spinal deformities in whom both supine and prone positioning are difficult. This position allows the protuberant abdomen and pannus to fall laterally, taking the weight off the anterior abdominal wall as occurs when the patient is supine. This maximizes diaphragmatic excursion and facilitates general anesthesia.

The lateral flexed position widens the space between the 12th rib and the iliac crest, flattening the folds of adipose tissue and facilitating percutaneous access.[2]

Advantages

1. Familiar to urologists who perform open renal surgery.
2. Easiest identification of the posterior calyces.
3. Useful in morbid obesity or severe kyphoscoliosis.
4. Least effect on cardiac and respiratory function.
5. Renal pelvis is dependent with easier access to mobile stones.
6. More ergonomic for the surgeon than prone position.
7. May perform nephroscopy and ureteroscopy simultaneously.

Disadvantages

1. Access can be achieved by ultrasound guidance or triangulation technique only with limited fluoroscopy range due to restricted arc of movement of the C-arm.
2. The ulnar nerve is at risk from the edge of the operating room table. The majority of these injuries can thus be prevented by adequate padding at the elbow and supination of the dependent arm.
3. Compression of the unpadded fibular head against the operating room (OR) table can result in peroneal nerve injury.

Randomized trials comparing flank to prone position and flank to supine to prone positions showed no difference in outcomes.[13]

COMPARISON OF RESULTS OF PCNL IN DIFFERENT POSITIONS

- The CROES PCNL Global Study analysed differences in patients' characteristics and perioperative outcomes between prone and supine PCNL from the database of 5775 patients. The operative time and stone-free rates favored prone PCNL, but patient safety favored supine PCNL. The authors concluded that choice of patient position should be tailored to individual patient characteristics and the surgeon's preference.[13]
- A prospective randomized study by Dessoukey et al concluded that PCNL in both positions was equally successful with no significant differences in complications. PCNL in the oblique supine lithotomy position was superior to PCNL in the prone position regarding operative time, hospital stay, and effects on respiratory and cardiovascular status (lower blood pressure, higher pulse rate and higher peak airway pressure in the prone position), making it more comfortable for patients and anesthesiologists. Morbidly obese patients, patients with cardiologic disorders, and patients with pulmonary obstructive airway disease may benefit from these differences.[14]
- With optimal placement of pads and bolsters, the prone position may provide better ventilation than the supine position.
- A recent meta-analysis by Patel RM, et al has shown a superior stone-free rate in the prone position and comparable complication rates to the supine position. The advantage of ease of access to the urethra for simultaneous retrograde techniques in the supine position is also possible with modifications in the prone position such as the split-leg technique.[15]
- Anatomical differences:[6] When the patient is positioned in the prone or prone-flexed positions, the spleen and liver rotate laterally, away from the kidney and nephrostomy tract, compared to when the patient is positioned supine (Fig. 3.3A). This would make it less likely that either of these organs would be injured with a puncture 30° from the vertical. In contrast, for lower pole punctures, the colon was more medially situated and more prone to injury in the prone and prone-flexed positions than when the patient was supine (Fig. 3.3B). The retrorenal colon is found on NCCT in 1.9% in the supine position compared with 10% in the prone position.[16]

CONCLUSION

Although both the supine and flank positions offer some potential benefits over prone positioning in certain settings, particularly morbid obesity and spinal deformities, the evidence suggests no overwhelming differences. Surgeon preference can determine the choice of position for percutaneous renal surgery.[17]

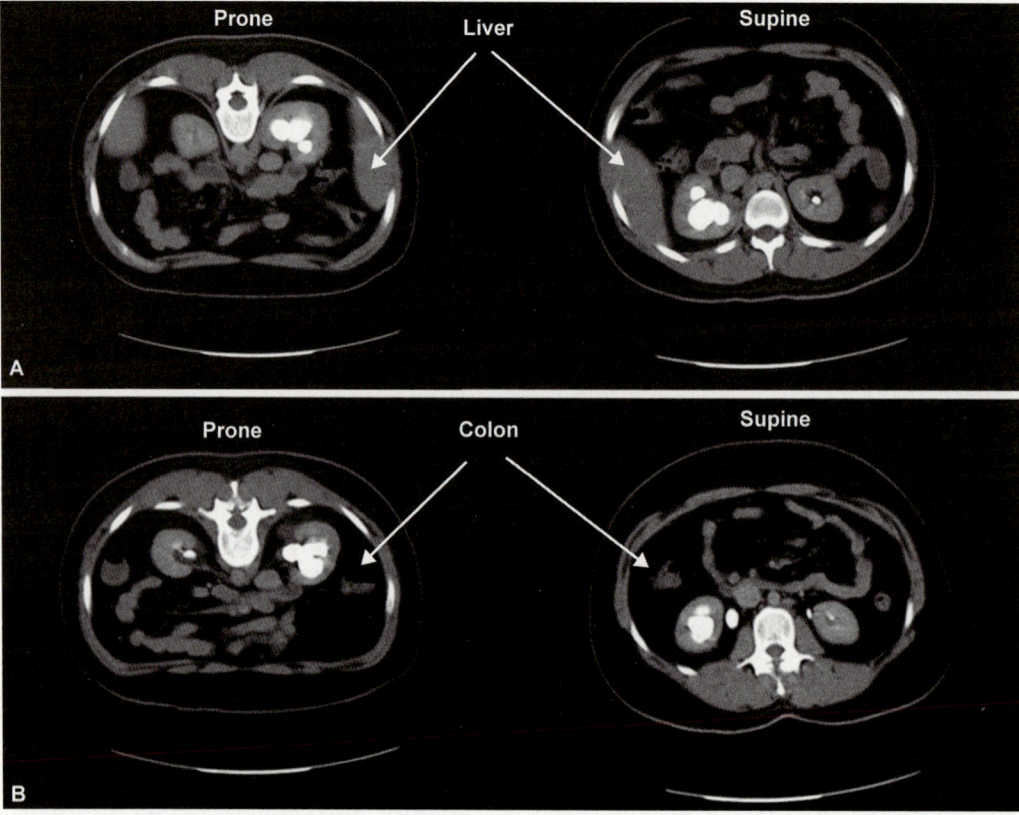

Fig. 3.3A and B: (A) Lateral rotation of liver and spleen in prone position; (B) Medial position of colon in prone position making it more prone to injury

References

1. J Stuart Wolf. Percutaneous Approaches to the Upper Urinary Tract Collecting System. Campbell-Walsh Urology, 11th edition.

2. Honey J and Ray AA. Prone, Lateral, and Flexed: Patient Positioning for Percutaneous Nephrolithotomy. Smith's Textbook of Endourology, third edition.

3. Bodin SG and Edwards AF. Special Anesthetic Considerations for Endourology: Ureteroscopy and Percutaneous Nephrolithotomy. Smith's Textbook of Endourology, third edition.

4. Chui J and Craen RA. An update on Prone position: Continuing Professional Development. Can J Anesth 2016;63:737–67.

5. Edgcombe, H., Carter, K., Yarrow, S. Anesthesia in the prone position. Br J Anaesth 2008;100:165–83.

6. Ray AA, Chung DG, Honey RJ. Percutaneous nephrolithotomy in the prone and prone-flexed positions: anatomic considerations. J Endourol 2009;23(10):1607–14.

7. Valdivia Uria JG. Patient Positioning for Supine Access. Smith's Textbook of Endourology, third edition.

8. Valdivia Uria JG, Valle Gerhold J, Lopez Lopez JA, et al. Technique and complications of percutaneous nephroscopy: experience with 557 patients in the supine position. J Urol 1998; 160:1975–88.

9. Kumar P, Bach C, Kachrilas S, et al. Supine percutaneous nephrolithotomy (PCNL): 'In vogue' but in which position? BJU Int 2012;110:1018–21.

10. Atkinson CJ, Turney BW, Noble JG, et al. Supine vs prone percutaneous nephrolithotomy: an anaesthetist's view. BJU Int 2011;108:306–08.

11. Duty B, Waingankar N, Okhunov Z, et al. Anatomical variation between the prone, supine,

and supine oblique positions on computed tomography: implications for percutaneous nephrolithotomy access. Urology 2012;79:67–71.

12. Kerbl K, Clayman RV, Chandhoke PS, et al. Percutaneous stone removal with the patient in a flank position. J Urol 1994;151:686–88.

13. Valdivia JG, Scarpa RM, Duvdevani M, et al. Supine versus prone position during percutaneous nephrolithotomy: a report from the clinical research office of the endourological society percutaneous nephrolithotomy global study. J Endourol 2011;25:1619–25.

14. Al-Dessoukey AA, Moussa AS, Abdelbary AM, et al. Percutaneous nephrolithotomy in the oblique supine lithotomy position and prone position: A comparative study. J Endourol 2014;28:1058–63.

15. Patel, R.M., Okhunov, Z., Clayman, R.V., et al. Prone versus supine percutaneous nephrolithotomy: What is your position? Curr Urol Rep 2017; 18: 26.

16. Hopper KD, Sherman JL, Luethke JM, Ghaed N. The retrorenal colon in the supine and prone patient. Radiology1987;162:443–46.

17. Karami H, Mohammadi R, Lotfi B. A study on comparative outcomes of percutaneous nephro-lithotomy in prone, supine, and flank positions. World J Urol 2013;31:1225–30.

SPINAL ANESTHESIA

All types of anesthesia have been used successfully for PCNL. This includes general, neuraxial, and local with sedation.[1] Traditionally general anesthesia (GA) has been the choice of anesthesia. GA, however has its own hazards like accidental extubation and kinking of endotracheal tube (ET) during prone positioning of the patient.

With increasing experience many urologists are now performing the procedure under spinal anesthesia.

NEURAL ANATOMY

Sympathetic innervation of the kidney arises from spinal segments T8 through L1 as preganglionic fibers that synapse in the celiac and aorticorenal ganglia, giving rise to the postsynaptic fibers that travel along the renal artery to reach their targets. Renal parasympathetic innervations are from vagal nerve fibers that also travel along the renal artery. The ureters receive their sympathetic input from spinal segments T10 to L2, and parasympathetics from S2 to S4 nerve roots. Painful stimuli from either distension or mucosal irritation will travel with the sympathetic fibers, as well as the ureters, to radiate up to the level of the upper kidney.[5] For this reason, any neuroaxial anesthetic should cover at least through sensory level T8.

This ensures that adequate anesthesia is provided several levels above the surgical site and that skin and chest wall sensory levels above the area where somatic stimulation will occur with instrumentation are also covered (T6).

Physiologic Effects[1]

- Cardiovascular effects include decrease in α_1 and β sympathetic stimulation effects ("sympathectomy") from the level of two to four dermatomes above the sensory block level achieved, leading to decreased blood pressure. Venous and arterial blood vessel tone both decrease. The decrease in venous return can cause a significant drop in cardiac output if the patient is volume depleted. Since cardiac perfusion is heavily dependent on diastolic filling pressure, a significant drop in MAP can have deleterious consequences in those with either significant coronary artery disease or low cardiac reserve.

- Pulmonary function: Tidal volumes are unchanged and vital capacity decreases slightly during SAB or epidural anesthesia as a result of paralysis of abdominal muscles. Those with severe respiratory compromise may suffer ineffective cough to clear secretions, due to paralysis of expiratory muscles.

Comparison between General and Spinal Anesthesia

- Interestingly, one randomized controlled trial demonstrated improved patient satisfaction, shorter postanesthesia care unit (PACU) times, and less postoperative pain through postoperative day 2, in 180 patients undergoing PCNL via combined spinal-epidural anesthesia versus GA.[2]
- Movasseghi and colleagues showed that patients undergoing PNCL under SA require smaller amounts of analgesic dose and show hemodynamic stability during surgery and recovery time. Also, SA technique provides decreased blood loss and shortened surgery as well as anesthesia times compared to GA.[3] They suggested that the reduced intra-thoracic pressure and epidural vein distension due to spontaneous ventilation results in reduced bleeding.
- In a large retrospective study, involving 1004 patients, complications were graded according to Clavien classification and comparison of the two groups was done which revealed that the overall rate of complications was greater in the GA group.[4]

Advantages

- Many of the issues related to positioning are resolved as the patients are conscious and can position himself/herself in the prone position according to their comfort.
- Reduced postoperative analgesia requirement.[5]

Disadvantages

- There is a risk of sudden hypotension after making the patient prone.
- Patient discomfort increases with the duration of the procedure and the surgeon may not feel comfortable in making skin punctures, especially those close to the 11th rib, if the patient is unable to coordinate breath holding at that time.

- A higher nephrostomy tract predisposes the patient to greater risk of incurring intrathoracic injury; therefore, when multiple or higher punctures are required to remove a greater stone load, GA would be safer and desirable. Vigilance is required throughout the procedure for raised airway pressures, end tidal CO_2 and falls in oxygen saturation indicating pleural or lung injury which should be managed promptly by maintaining ventilation with 100% oxygen and if pneumothorax is diagnosed intraoperatively, by placement of chest tube.[5]

CONCLUSION

- Complexity of procedure, surgeon preference and patient co-morbidities are the factors to be considered when planning the anesthesia for PCNL.
- Complex stones like large bulk or staghorn calculus, upper calyceal calculi necessitating supracostal puncture, low surgeon experience, pediatric procedure and patient co-morbidities like poor cardiac reserve and apprehensive patients would necessitate general anesthesia.

References

1. Bodin SG and Edwards AF. Special Anesthetic Considerations for Endourology: Ureteroscopy and Percutaneous Nephrolithotomy. Smith's Textbook of Endourology, third edition.

2. Karacalar, S., Bilen, C.Y., Sarihasan, B. et al. Spinal-epidural anesthesia versus general anesthesia in the management of percutaneous nephrolithotripsy. J Endourol 2009;23:1591–97.

3. Movasseghi G, et al. Comparison Between Spinal and General Anesthesia in Percutaneous Nephrolithotomy. Anesth Pain Med 2014 Feb; 4(1): e13871.

4. T. Cicek, U. Gonulalan, R. Dogan, et al. "Spinal anesthesia is an efficient and safe anesthetic method for percutaneous nephrolithotomy." Urology 2014;83(1):50–55.

5. Indira Malik and Rachna Wadhwa, "Percutaneous Nephrolithotomy: Current Clinical Opinions and Anesthesiologists Perspective," Anesthesiology Research and Practice, 2016.

4 Tract Dilatation

Rajesh Kukreja

Tract dilation is an essential step in the performance of percutaneous renal surgery. With proper tract dilation, an appropriate size working sheath can then be placed, facilitating the insertion of the endoscopes, working instruments, and nephrostomy tube. Dilatation is always performed over a guidewire.

Placing a Secured Guidewire

Establishing a secure wire is the key to successful tract dilatation and PCNL.

- Free flow of saline or urine from the 18 gauge needle confirms a correct puncture.
- A 0.038 or 0.035 inch hydrophilic nitinol core glidewire is then passed through the needle and into the collecting system. The nitinol core glidewire is preferred because it is quite maneuverable and resists kinking (Fig. 4.1A). If a 21-gauge puncture needle that accepts a 0.018-inch wire has been used, transition dilators are necessary to upsize to a larger working wire.[1, 2]
- Under fluoroscopic guidance an attempt is made to advance the glidewire down the ureter. If the wire does not pass easily into the ureter, it can be coiled in the renal pelvis.
- Maneuvers to negotiate the wire into the ureter include:
  - An 8 Fr fascial dilator is passed into the calyx, followed by a 5 Fr Cobra tipped angiographic catheter. The angiographic catheter helps direct the glidewire towards the ureteropelvic junction (UPJ), facilitating placement of the wire down the ureter.
  - With help of a stiff dilator like an Alken rod, the kidney can be tented cephalad. This helps in straightening any kink at the ureter or UPJ and negotiating the glidewire across. This maneuver is especially helpful in lower calyceal punctures at acute angle to the ureter.
- After the glidewire is positioned in the ureter it may be exchanged for a stiffer, polytetrafluoroethylene coated working wire, such as a Zebra or Amplatz super-stiff wire (Fig. 4.1B). The lubricious nature of the glidewire makes it prone to displacement.
- An 8/10 Fr coaxial dilator or the dilatation cannula (Karl Storz) (Fig. 4.2) is used to place a second safety wire, usually a 0.035-inch wire. For beginners, it is imperative to have a safety wire in place before proceeding with percutaneous tract dilation.

Methods of Tract Dilatation

Several methods of tract dilatation are available, including metal telescoping dilators, semirigid Amplatz dilators and balloon dilators.

A. Alken's Dilators

These are rigid telescoping metal stainless steel dilators that are introduced over a central guide rod.[3] Progressively enlarging and

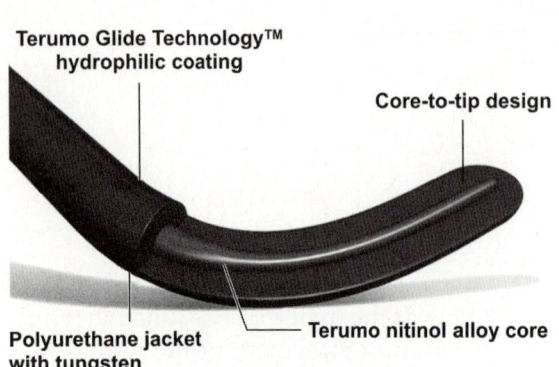

Terumo Glide Technology™
hydrophilic coating

Core-to-tip design

Polyurethane jacket
with tungsten

Terumo nitinol alloy core

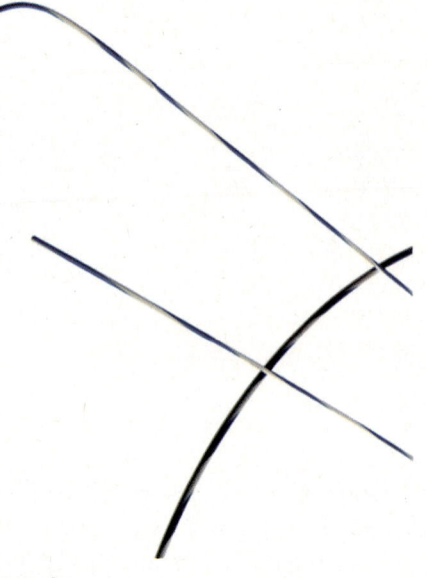

(A) Nitinol core hydrophilic guidewire
- Core: Nitinol core for flexibility and shape memory
- Coating: Polyurethane coating for smooth soft surface has tungsten added for radio-opacity
- Hydrophilic material (M polymer): Causes water to stick on surface making it smooth and slippery.
- Diameter (Inch): 0.018, 0.025, 0.035 and 0.038
- Lengths: 80, 150, 180 and 260 cm
- 3 cm floppy tip: Straight/angle/J tip

(B) Zebra wire
- Kink resistant nitinol core with flexible PTFE jacket for torque ability
- Blue and white striped pattern for better endoscopic visualization and handling
- Platinum distal tip: Visible under fluoroscopy
- Lubricious uro-glide coating on distal 60 cm to reduce friction and make it kink resistant like a glidewire
- Advantages of both guidewire and glidewire and disadvantage of none

Fig. 4.1A and B: Guidewires. (A) Nitinol core hydrophilic guidewire; (B) Zebra wire

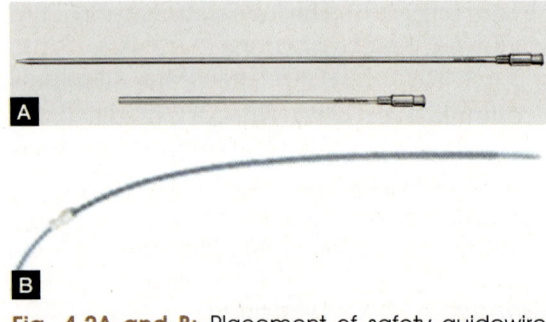

A

B

Fig. 4.2A and B: Placement of safety guidewire. (A) 3 mm dilatation cannula (set of inner and outer cannula) (Karl Storz); (B) 8 Fr (70 cm long) Stylet with 10 Fr (30 cm long) introducer sheath; PTFE; kink resistant (Boston Scientific)

telescoping coaxial stainless steel dilators starting from 9 Fr with successive increments of 3 Fr help to dilate the tract from the 7 Fr hollow guide rod up to 30 Fr (Fig. 4.3). The

Rough surface
for hand grip

Assembled dilators

Knob at the
tip of the rod

Outermost
dilator

Central
rod

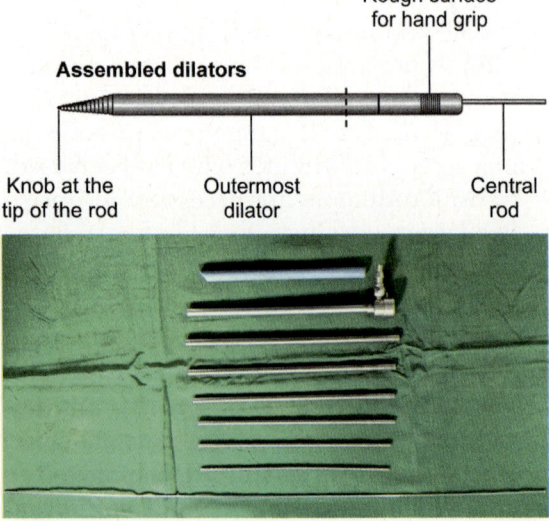

Fig. 4.3: Alken telescoping coaxial stainless steel dilators

guide rod (7 Fr) has a round bulbous end (9 Fr) that prevents the sequential dilators from overshooting.[4] The advantages of the Alken's dilator system are that it is reusable, hence inexpensive and importantly is able to dilate even when there is dense perinephric scarring. The ability of these dilators to dilate right till their ends is useful in difficult situations like a complete staghorn with minimal space between the calyceal wall and the edge of stone.

The disadvantage is that the same characteristics that make the Alken's dilator so effective are also the reasons why the rigid metal dilators can do considerable damage. They have an increased potential for iatrogenic injury, due to difficulty with controlling the pressure during dilation. Moreover, the necessity for manual stabilization of the central rod during the dilation increases the risk of perforating the renal pelvis.

B. *Amplatz Dilators*

These are semi rigid tapered-tip polyurethane cylindrical dilators, of progressively increasing circumference, ranging from 8 to 30 F that are passed over an 8 Fr angiographic catheter that fits over a 0.035-inch guidewire (Fig. 4.4).[5] They can also be passed over the Alken's guide rod. The dilators are passed one after the other, not coaxially like the rigid metal dilators but progressively, by advancing one dilator, removing it, advancing the next larger dilator, and so on until the final tract diameter is achieved. Finally, the working sheath is passed over the final dilator and then the dilator and 8 Fr catheter are removed, leaving the working wire and sheath in place. The dilators are made in increments of 2 Fr, but if the tissue being dilated is soft, then not every dilator needs to be used.

The advantages of Amplatz dilators are that trauma experienced by the collecting system is theoretically less than the trauma experienced by the collecting system using rigid metal dilators, but the disadvantage is that bleeding can happen each time a dilator is withdrawn. As these are disposable dilators, they are more expensive than the Alken's dilators.

There have been many comparative studies between the two dilator systems but experienced urologists have found no difference between the two systems in terms of safety. Alken's dilators may be preferred in patients who have a tight fitting staghorn calculus, as Amplatz dilators need some space in the calyx for dilatation. The shoulder or the tapered end of each Amplatz dilator must be advanced entirely within the entry calyx. In calyces that have no space, the dilatation may remain short due to tapered end of the dilator.

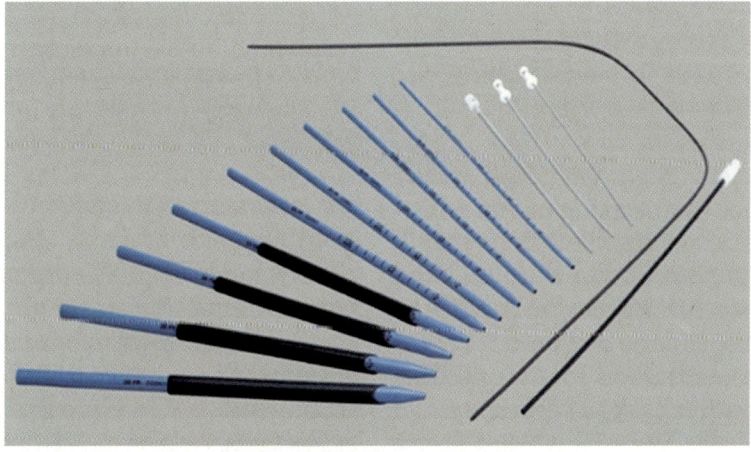

Fig. 4.4: Amplatz dilator set

C. Balloon Dilators

The balloon dilator set consists of an expandable balloon, a working Amplatz sheath that is back-loaded before the inflated balloon is placed over the wire, and syringe inflator.[1] The balloon comes in inflated balloon diameters of 6, 8 and 10 mm with length of 15 cm and transparent or PTFE sheaths (Fig. 4.5) (Ultraxx, Cook Medical). Pressures of up to 20 atmospheres can be easily achieved with this system, although in general, much lower pressures are usually sufficient for tract creation. Balloon inflation is performed using radiographic contrast instilled within the injector syringe. The balloon should be inflated until no "waisting" or focal narrowing is evident. The pressure required to dilate the tract is generally under 15 cm H_2O. The balloon dilator should be manually stabilized during this procedure in order to avoid inadvertent displacement. Balloon inflation allows for full expansion of the balloon, which is followed by insertion of a working sheath over the balloon, in a rotational manner.

Balloon dilators have been reported to cause significantly less bleeding than sequential dilators because the radial force used to spread the renal parenchyma is less traumatic than the shearing or cutting action of sequential Amplatz dilators or metal telescoping dilators. The main disadvantage of the balloon dilator system is the cost. Sequential Amplatz or metal dilators may be useful in the setting of extensive perirenal fibrosis from previous renal surgery. However, an X-Force™ N30 nephrostomy balloon dilation catheter (Bard Urological, Covington, Georgia) can achieve 30 atmospheres. This may prove advantageous in the presence of flank scarring.[2] Alternatively a 4.5 mm fascial incising needle (Fig. 4.6) (Cook Urological, Spencer, Indiana) can be placed over the working wire to facilitate balloon dilation.

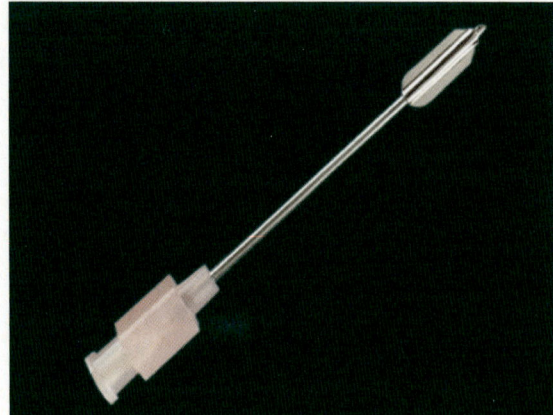

Fig. 4.6: Cook fascia incising needle

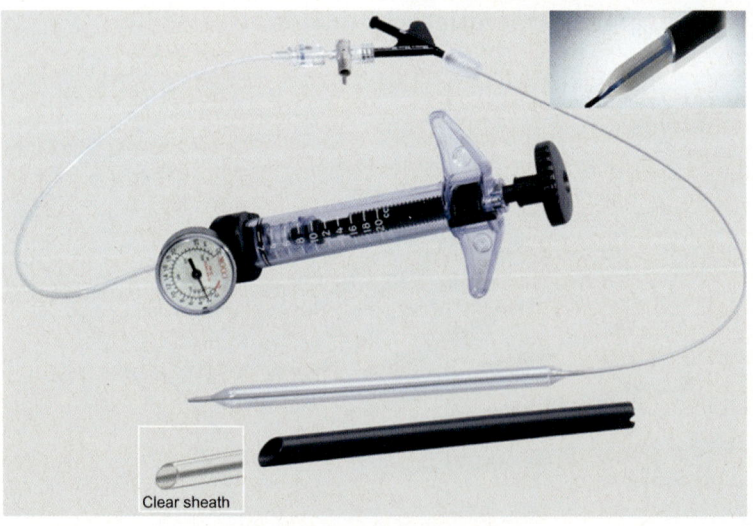

Clear sheath

Fig. 4.5: Balloon dilator set

D. *Single Step Dilatation*

In an effort to make tract making rapid, easy, and blood less, multiple single step techniques have been described.

- The simplest is using the largest Amplatz dilators without the initial smaller dilators.
- Screw dilators: These have a screw-shaped tapered conical tip (Fig. 4.7). They are available in 3 sizes—size 6 to 12 Fr, 6 to 14 Fr and 6 to 16 Fr (6 implies the size of tip and 12 implies the size of the shaft).
- The miniaturised PCNL sets have their own single step dilators (Fig. 4.8).

Two new dilatation systems described have been a radially expanding single step dilator system[6] and the 5-PANG system (Fig. 4.9).[7] Both the systems offer the advantage of not removing the needle and hence the dilatation is over s rigid system resulting in less chances of kinking of guidewire. Also the dilatation would be faster.

There have been many comparative studies between the dilator systems but no significant difference has been found between all the systems in terms of safety.[8–13]

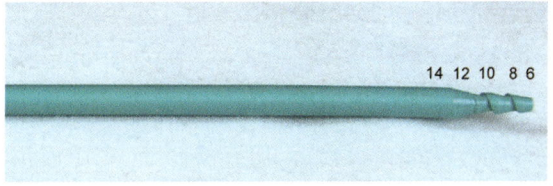

Fig. 4.7: Single step screw dilator

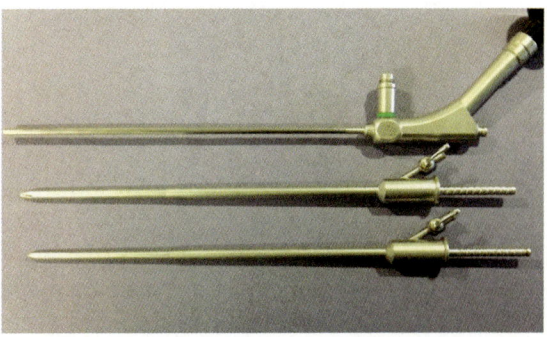

Fig. 4.8: Nagele Modular MIP System (Storz): Each Mini PERC sheath has its own single step dilator to be passed over the wire directly with the sheath back-loaded over its dilator

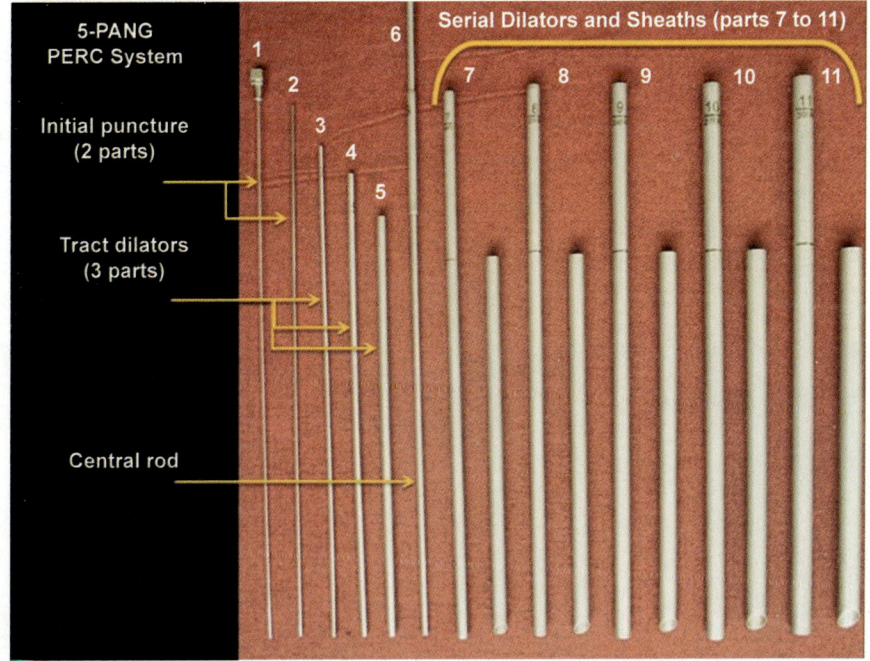

Fig. 4.9: 5-PANG System: Set of telescoping dilators with advantage of not removing the puncture needle hence avoiding chances of kinking the wire

Principles of Tract Dilatation

Whatever may be the mode of tract dilatation, certain principles need to be strictly adhered to.[8, 14]

- The success of tract dilatation is dependent on maintaining the angle, depth, and the direction of the dilatation.
- Every step of dilatation should be monitored on fluoroscopy.
- The lumbodorsal fascia should be incised with a sharp blade knife passed along the needle under fluoroscopic guidance as a lumbotome or the 18 G Cook fascia incising needle (Fig. 4.6) passed over the wire. The fascia should be incised in two planes at right angles to each other. The fascia is the site of greatest resistance to the dilatation. This maneuver is especially helpful in case with retroperitoneal scarring and fibrosis due to previous surgeries. Care should be taken to avoid lacerating the nearby subcostal or intercostal neurovascular bundle on the inferior rib margin.
- The tract should be dilated only till the minor calyx. If overdilatation happens, it can traumatize the infundibulum, renal pelvis or ureteropelvic junction. Trauma to the anterior wall of the PCS can cause significant bleeding that may be difficult to control. It is always better to underdilate than to overdilate and cause trauma.
- Each dilator should be passed in the same phase of respiration as was during the puncture.

- Dilatation should always be rotating movements at the wrist joint (alternating supination and pronation) with minimal forward thrust. Attempt should be to dilate till the calyx and not till the calculus.
- The collecting system should be kept distended during dilatation by constant saline flushing through the retrograde ureteric catheter by the OR assistant. Free exit of the flushed saline from the dilators confirms entry of the dilator into the pelvicalyceal system (Fig. 4.10).
- Guidewire friction test: Ridhorkar et al demonstrated that free to and fro movements of the guidewire after every step of sequential dilatation indicates well aligned dilatation without kinking of the guidewire.[15] Lack of free flow of saline through the dilators or presence of a kinked guidewire as confirmed by the guidewire friction test indicate improper dilatation due to wrong direction or angle of dilatation.
- Difficult conditions like retroperitoneal scarring or obesity are risk factors for guidewire kinking and loss of plane of dilatation.

Complications of Renal Tract Dilatation

A. Hemorrhage: Acute hemorrhage can originate from either of these four sources: Intercostal vessels, renal parenchymal vasculature, branches of the renal vein and renal artery adjacent to the pelvicalyceal system. The reported incidence of serious arterial injuries ranges from 0.9 to 3% after percutaneous

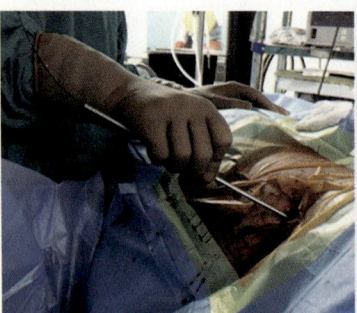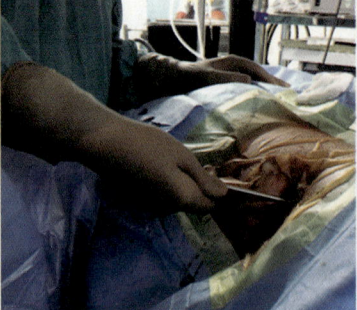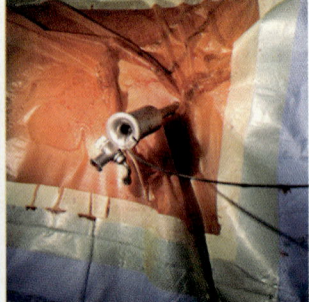

Fig. 4.10: Dilatation: Alternate pronation and supination movements of the forearm without any forward thrusting movements. Clear flow of saline from the sheath indicates well placed and nontraumatic dilatation

procedures.[1, 10, 12] The most clinically significant bleeding related to percutaneous tract dilation is due to over-advancement of the dilating instrument, resulting in splitting of the infundibulum. This occurrence can be avoided by understanding the anatomy of the entry calyx and infundibulum with retrograde contrast injection. Regardless of the dilating system used, the intention should then be to place the widest part of the dilator into the entry calyx, but not into the infundibulum.

B. Renal pelvis perforation: The most common cause of renal pelvis perforation is the aggressive use of serial dilators. The perforation is usually medial, following an over-advancement of the dilator. Renal pelvis perforation can also occur due to initial transgression of the puncture needle and in appropriate guidewire positioning. Initial advancement of the guidewire down the ureter and into the bladder facilitates dilation and greatly reduces the risk of this complication. The perforation is usually recognized intraoperatively by visualization of perinephric or renal sinus fat and contrast extravasation on fluoroscopy. Once recognized, it may require quick termination of the procedure and placement of a ureteral stent and a nephrostomy tube.

TROUBLESHOOTING DURING DILATATION

Underdilated Tract

- **Identification**
  - There is no free flow of saline from the exterior end of Amplatz sheath. Instead, hemorrhagic efflux is seen.
  - On passing the nephroscope, we see fat with the distal end of Amplatz sheath outside the pelvicalyceal system.
- **Cause:** This usually occurs early during the learning curve. Use of Amplatz dilators is associated with this as the terminal taper end of the dilator enters the calyx but the Amplatz sheath introduced over, it does not

enter the calyx and remains outside the collecting system. This may cause brisk bleeding as there is a portion of parenchyma that has been partially dilated, which does not have the tamponade effects of the Amplatz sheath.

- **Prevention**
  - The collecting system should be kept distended during dilatation by constant saline flushing through the retrograde ureteric catheter by the OR assistant. Free exit of the flushed saline from the dilators and the Amplatz sheath confirms entry of the dilator into the pelvicalyceal system.
  - When using the Amplatz dilators, you need to pass the dilator well into the system so that the dilator beyond the terminal tapered segment has entered the calyx.
- **Solution**
  - Load the guide rod and Amplatz dilator corresponding to the sheath size over the guidewire. Pass the guide rod over the wire into the calyx and the dilator over the rod. Entry into the system is identified by free flow of flushed saline. Now reposition the sheath over the dilator.
  - If the wire has slipped out of the system, you may flush dilute betadine or methylene blue from the ureteric catheter and identify the opening in the renal parenchyma under nephroscopic vision. Pass the wire through the identified rent from where you can see betadine or methylene blue coming out. The wire should enter the pelvicalyceal system. Re-dilate now over the wire.
  - If this too fails, a new puncture may be required. This may be difficult as the contrast may extravasate or the calyx may not fill due to leakage of contrast. Choosing an access through another calyx or sonography-guided puncture may help.

– In a rare situation, it may be needed to stage the procedure. The puncture site seals in 48–72 hours and a repeat procedure can be done after that time.

Overdilatation

- **Identification**
  – On passing the nephroscope, we see fat with the distal end of Amplatz sheath outside the pelvicalyceal system.
- **Cause:** Overdilatation is a state when the dilators have traversed the opposite wall of the PCS and the Amplatz sheath is now placed anterior to the kidney. Forceful dilatation is the usual reason for this problem.
- **Prevention:** Dilatation should always be by rotating movements at the wrist joint (alternating supination and pronation) with minimal forward thrust. Attempt should be to dilate till the calyx and not till the calculus.
- **Solution (Fig. 4.11)**
  – The Amplatz sheath needs to be withdrawn back to get it in the PCS. The perforated pelvic wall will not have any tamponade effect and may bleed. Also, the irrigation fluid would leak through the hole and may cause significant fluid overload. Even the stone or stone fragments can migrate outside the PCS through the hole in the anterior wall.
  – The further plan after this would depend on the size of perforation, size of the stone and the amount of bleeding.

– If the size of the perforation and the stone both are small, than one can get back properly in the system and quickly finish the procedure without causing much extravasation.

– However, if there is a large perforation or a large stone or significant bleeding than it is prudent to insert a nephrostomy tube, abandon the procedure. Always keep a large bore nephrostomy tube during such situations. The second procedure can be staged after 2 or 3 days, as the perforation usually heals during this period.

Kinking of Guidewire

- **Cause:** This usually occurs due to forceful dilatation in the wrong direction. This is like to occur when the tract is not in a straight line. Retrorenal fibrosis, obesity and an oblique or acutely angulated tract are risk factors. Once the guide rod is in place this problem cannot occur.
- **Prevention**
  – The wire usually kinks at the level of the thoracolumbar fascia. Hence, the fascia needs to be incised well before starting the dilatation.
  – Dilatation should always be rotating movements at the wrist joint (alternating supination and pronation) with minimal forward thrust.
  – If there is doubt regarding the correct direction then moving the glidewire

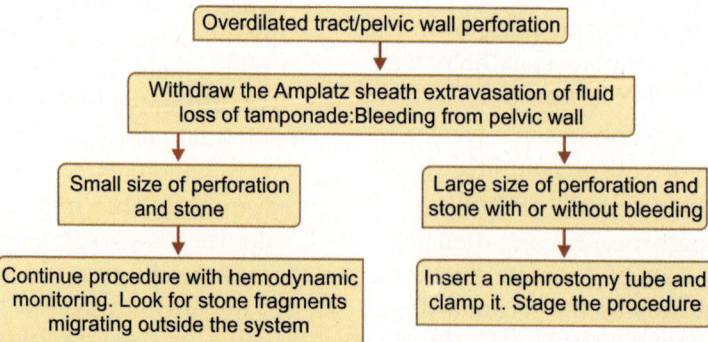

Fig. 4.11: Algorithm for management of overdilated tract and pelvic wall perforation

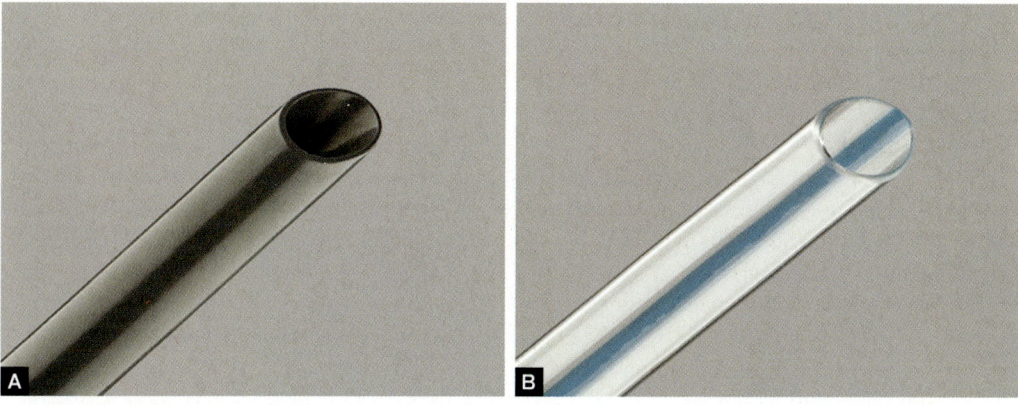

Fig. 4.12A and B: Amplatz sheath. (A) Opaque sheath; (B) Clear with radiopaque stripe

(friction test) gives a good indication. If the wire moves freely then it indicates that the direction and trajectory is correct. Vice versa, if the glidewire does not move freely then the direction and trajectory needs to be adjusted.

– Each dilator should be passed in the same phase of respiration was during the puncture.

– Use of the 5 part PANG needle system largely avoids this problem.[7]

• **Solution**
  – If a kink has occurred then the initial dilator should be advanced close to the kink and the kinked portion of guidewire pulled inside the dilator. The correct direction should then be ascertained and further dilation should be done. Once the initial dilator (6 or 8 Fr) is inside the kidney, replace the wire with a new one.
  – At times a re-puncture is needed.
  – If a safety wire has been inserted then it can be used for dilatation.

AMPLATZ SHEATH

No matter the type of dilator used, rigid or balloon, or the technique of track dilation, one-step or multi-stepped, an Amplatz sheath is always used for a standard PCNL. These are available in sizes ranging from 12 to 34 Fr with length ranging from 16 to 30 cm (Cook Medical). Opaque or clear sheath with radiopaque stripes are available (Fig. 4.12).

Benefits of an Amplatz Sheath

1. Amplatz sheath maintains the tract during procedure.
2. It causes tamponade of the tract and reduces bleeding. The beveled end of the Amplatz sheath can be used to tamponade a part of renal parenchyma that is actively bleeding.
3. It protects the renal parenchyma from injury by the instruments used in renal procedures.
4. The use of Amplatz sheath maintains a low-pressure system and reduces fluid intravasation. Maintaining a low-pressure system would be important in patients with infected calculi as the risk of sepsis would reduce.

Care should be taken to avoid over- or under-advancement of the sheath on the dilators because this may cause bleeding and trauma to the renal parenchyma or collecting system.

References

1. Petar Erdeljan, Hassan Razvi. Dilation of the Nephrostomy Tract. Smith's Textbook of Endourology. 3rd edn.
2. Miller NL, Matlaga BR, Lingeman JE. Techniques for fluoroscopic percutaneous renal access. J Urol 2007;178:15–23.

3. Alken P. The telescope dilators. World J Urol. 1985;3:7–10.

4. Knoll, T., Michael, M.S. Alken, P. Surgical Atlas. Percutaneous nephrolithotomy: the Mennheim technique. BJU Int 2007;99:213–31.

5. Rusnak B, Castañeda-Zúñiga W, Kotula F, et al. An improved dilator system for percutaneous nephrostomies. Radiology. 1982;144:174.

6. Goharderakhshan RZ, Schwartz BF, Rudnick DM, Irby PB, Stoller ML. Radially expanding single-step nephrostomy tract dilator. Urology 2001; 58: 693–96.

7. Patil AV. A novel 5-part Percutaneous Access Needle with Glidewire technique (5-PANG) for percutaneous nephrolithotomy: our initial experience. Urology 2010; 75.

8. Sharma GR, Maheshwari PN, Sharma AG, Maheshwari RP, Heda RS, Maheshwari SP. Fluoro-scopy-guided percutaneous renal access in prone position. World J Clin Cases 2015;3(3): 245–64.

9. Davidoff R, Bellman GC. Influence of technique of percutaneous tract creation on incidence of renal hemorrhage. J Urol 1997;157:1229–31.

10. Safak, M., Gogus, C., Soygur, T. Nephrostomy tract dilation using a balloon dilator in percutaneous renal surgery:experience with 95 cases and comparison with the fascial dilator system. Urol Int 2003;71:382–84.

11. Al-Kandari, A.M., Jabbour, M., Anderson, A. et al. Comparative study of degree of renal trauma between Amplatz sequential fascial dilation and balloon dilation during percutaneous renal surgery in an animal model. Urology 2007;69:586–89.

12. Gonen, M., Istanbulluoglu, O.M. Cicek, T et al. Balloon dilatation versus Amplatz dilatation for nephrostomy tract dilatation. J Endourol 2008; 22:901–04.

13. Dehong C, Liangren L, Huawei L, Qiang W. A comparison among four tract dilation methods of percutaneous nephrolithotomy:A systematic review and meta-analysis. Urolithiasis 2013; 41:523–30.

14. Wolf JS. Percutaneous approaches to the upper urinary tract collecting system. Campbell-Walsh Urology. 10th edn. Philadelphia,PA: Saunders Elsevier, 2011.

15. Ridhorkar VR, Desai RM, Sabnis RB, et al. Guide-wire friction test: an aid to PCNL tract dilatation. Indian J Urol 1998;14:74–76.

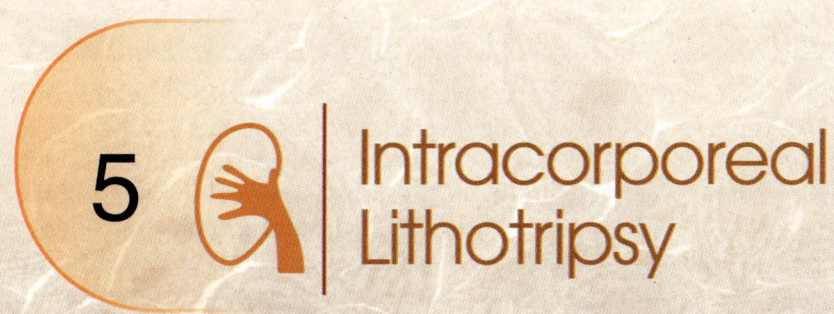

5 | Intracorporeal Lithotripsy

Rajesh Kukreja

Currently, percutaneous nephrolithotomy (PCNL) employs four techniques for intracorporeal lithotripsy in clinical practice: Electrohydraulic lithotripsy (EHL), ultrasonic lithotripsy, pneumatic lithotripsy, and laser lithotripsy (Table 5.1). Each of these lithotripsy devices has inherent benefits and limitations to their utilization.

Table 5.1: Types of energy sources				
	Ultrasonic	*Pneumatic*	*Electrohydraulic*	*Holmium laser*
Mechanism of action	Piezoceramic crystals: Rapid probe vibrations: mechanical fracture of stone	Ballistic tip; kinetic energy: Jackhammer action	Electric spark with shock waves	Thermal drilling/ melting with weak shock waves
Probe distance from stone	In contact	In contact	Very close (1–2 mm) to stone	In contact
Suction	Present	Option (Lithovac)	Absent	Options available
Probe distance from lens	No effect	No effect	2–5 mm at least	2 mm beyond the lens
Probe/fiber sizes	2.5–12 Fr	0.8–2.5 mm	1.9–3.3 Fr	200–1000 µm
Flexible probes	Absent	Absent	Present	Present
Tissue effects	Potential for thermal injury, if irrigation is interrupted Mucosal stripping	Least traumatic amongst all Focal areas of hemorrhage and mucosal erosions	Energy <500 mJ/ pulse: No histologic damage Energy = 1000 mJ: 1 cm longitudinal ureteric perforation	Safe provided the distance between the tip of the fiber and mucosa is >1 mm
Fragment retropulsion	Low due to suction	Present, can be reduced by lithovac	Present	Minimal
Effect of stone composition	Nil	Effective for hard stones, less efficient for soft stones	Present; weakest efficiency in uric acid stones	Nil

ELECTROHYDRAULIC LITHOTRIPSY

Invented by Yutkin in 1955, EHL was first put to use by Rouvalis in 1970 in a series of 100 patients of bladder stones.[1]

Mechanism of action of the EHL probe is that of an underwater spark plug. The probe consists of two separate concentric electrodes of different voltage polarities. As current is applied, the resistance of the insulative gap eventually is overcome and a spark is produced. This spark in turn vaporizes the surrounding fluid, creating a cavitation bubble that expands and subsequently collapses.[2] A total of three shock waves are created through the process of rapid expansion, collapse, and rebound of the cavitation bubble.[3] Therefore, if the probe is held in direct contact with the stone, minimal water is vaporized and an in efficient shock wave is created. Technically, the EHL probe should be held approximately 1 mm from the stone to allow for maximal effect and at least 2–5 mm from the lens of the scope to prevent instrument damage.

Probes between 1.9 and 3.3 Fr are available. Thinner probes are considered more versatile because of their application in flexible and semirigid ureteroscopy. Reducing probe diameter does not clearly lessen fragmentation potential; however, durability is decreased. Pressure generated by EHL probes is estimated using the formula: Maximum pressure = energy/(pulse duration × fiber cross sectional diameter).

Tissue Effects

Vorreuther and colleagues attempted to quantify tissue damage resulting from the use of a 3.3 Fr Wolf EHL probe.[4] Using freshly harvested human ureters, histologic changes were measured after direct contact with the EHL probe. At 100 mJ, only punctate mucosal injuries were noted, whereas increasing to 400 to 600 mJ caused superficial mechanical defects in the muscularis. Increasing the energy to 1000 mJ caused transmural perforations. Microscopically, no thermal injuries were noted, and defects appeared to be due to mechanical disruptions, although limited to the cross-sectional diameter of the probe. When maintaining constant energy levels, altering voltage and/or capacity did not affect the resulting histologic findings. No damage was encountered at a distance of 1 mm between the probe tip and mucosa, even at maximal energy and pulse rates. When tested in an intact ureter, the probe tip was centered in the lumen, and no histologic damage was encountered at energy settings less than 500 mJ/pulse. When energy levels reached 1000 mJ, a single pulse could produce a 1 cm longitudinal ureteric perforation. Thought to be secondary to cavitation bubbles, which can reach 1.5 cm in diameter at greater than 1300 mJ, the rapid expansion effectively burst the ureter.

Disadvantages and Limitations

1. Ureteral perforation: In clinical practice, the development of smaller EHL probes has improved clinical safety. Overall, ureteral perforation is noted to have a mean incidence of 8.5%.[5]

2. Another disadvantage of EHL is its propensity to propel fragments, as well as to create an ample number of fragments when large (>15 mm) stones are treated. In a series of 43 patients with a single ureteral stone proximal to the pelvic brim treated with EHL, 14% required subsequent ESWL to treat stones that had been inadvertently pushed into the renal pelvis.[6]

3. Chemical stone composition has been shown to affect fragmentation efficiency during EHL ureteroscopy. A review of operating room times for 193 patients was compared with the chemical composition of ureteric stones. Uric acid stones required the most time, followed by calcium oxalate monohydrate, and in multivariate analysis,

stone size was negatively associated with successful fragmentation.[7] This association may be due to the smooth outer surface and lamination of uric acid stones being more difficult for shockwave-generated fragmentation.

Advantage

Smaller probes are flexible enough to allow their use with flexible ureteroscopes. In a series of 207 ureteral and renal stones treated with EHL, 90.3% were successfully fragmented with an 82.1% stone free rate at 20 months follow-up.[8] Similarly, Green and Lytton reported excellent fragmentation of 32 of 36 stones with the use of a 5F EHL probe.[4] Overall, the literature demonstrates a mean 90% fragmentation rate for ureteral stones treated with EHL.[5]

References

1. Rouvalis, P. Electronic lithotripsy for vesical calculus with "Urat-1". An experience of 100 cases and an experimental application of the method to stones in the upper urinary tract. Br J Urol 1970;42:486–91.

2. Grocela, J.A., Dretler, S.P. Intracorporeal lithotripsy. Instrumentation and development. Urol Clin North Am 1997;24:13–23.

3. Zhong, P., Tong, H.L., Cocks, F.H., Preminger, G.M. Transient oscillation of cavitation bubbles near stone surface during electrohydraulic lithotripsy. J Endourol1997;11:55–61.

4. Vorreuther R, Corleis R, Klotz T, et al. Impact of shock wave pattern and cavitation bubble size on tissue damage during ureteroscopic electrohydraulic lithotripsy. J Urol 1995;153 (3 Pt 1):849–53.

5. Lingeman, J.E., Matlaga, B.R., Evan, A.P. Surgical management of upper urinary tract calculi. In: Wein, A.J., Kavoussum L.R., Novick, A.C., Partin, A.W., Peters, C.A.,eds. Campbell-Walsh Urology, 9th edn, Philadelphia: WB Saunders, 2007, pp. 1431–506.

6. Yang, S.S., Hong, J.S. Electrohydraulic lithotripsy of upper ureteral calculi with semirigid ureteroscope. J Endourol 1996;10:27–30.

7. Song HC, Jung HB, Lee YS, et al. Influence of ureteral stone components on the outcomes of electrohydraulic lithotripsy. Korean J Urol 2012;53:848–52.

8. Basar, H., Ohta, N., Kageyama, S., Suzuki, K., Kawabe, K. Treatment of ureteral and renal stones by electrohydraulic lithotripsy. Int Urol Nephrol 1997; 29:275–80.

ULTRASONIC LITHOTRIPSY

The upper limit of sound audible to the human ear is generally regarded to be 20 kHz. Sound waves with a frequency above this threshold are referred to as ultrasound waves.

Mechanism of Action

Ultrasonic lithotrites pass electrical current through piezoceramic crystals, producing directional sound waves of 23,000 to 27,000 Hz. The handpiece houses, the piezoelectric interface, and waves propagate as mechanical vibrational energy longitudinally down a solid or metal probe to where contact is made with the stone.[1] As the metal probe vibrates, when contact is made with the stone, this reverberation transmitted to the stone causes fracturing along with the mechanical trauma of the oscillating metal tip against the surface.

Solid metal probes disintegrate stones by transmitting mechanical energy in a transverse plane, rather than longitudinally as with hollow probes. Local fracture can produce fine debris, which is aspirated by the probe; or if the probe is applied to fault lines, regional breakage can be created leading to larger fragments. As the mechanism of stone fragmentation in ultrasonic lithotripsy is purely mechanical, direct contact with the stone is necessary.[2]

Probes

Ultrasonic probes are manufactured in a variety of sizes from 2.5 to 12 F. The larger probes incorporate a hollow channel through which suction is applied [the smaller probes (2.5 F) are solid in design and therefore, lack suction]. The presence of this channel gives these devices a major advantage in that small stone fragments (<2 mm) can be evacuated as lithotripsy is performed.

Tissue Effects

Piergiovanni et al studied the effect of EHL, ultrasonic, pneumatic, and laser lithotripsy on pig bladder and ureteral tissues and demonstrated that perforation was not possible with ultrasonic or pneumatic lithotripsy. These animals were sacrificed on days 0, 1, and 6. Histologic examination demonstrated that injury was limited to abrasions of the epithelium.[3] These authors concluded that ultrasound and pneumatic lithotripsy are safer than EHL and laser lithotripsy.

The mechanism of stone destruction raises a concern regarding the generation of heat at the site of interaction between the stone and probe. Although there is a potential for thermal injury, it is only of concern if irrigation is interrupted, as it has been demonstrated that at an irrigation rate of 30 ml/min, the change in temperature at the probe tip is minimal (1.4°C).[4]

Uses

PCNL: Ultrasonic lithotripsy has found its greatest utility in PCNL. The nephroscope's large caliber allows for the utilization of larger probes with a greater ability to evacuate stone fragments. Many researchers have demonstrated percutaneous ultrasonic treatment of large renal stones to be an effective and safe procedure with success rates of 80.4–100%.[5, 6]

Larger pieces can be fragmented further or extracted manually. Using continuous irrigation and suction keep the probe tip cool, while continuously removing particles. As the fluid is evacuated through the handpiece, it cools the piezoceramic crystals, which can rapidly increase in temperature if proper suction is not maintained. Without adequate suction, in addition to a noticeably hot handpiece, visualization and stone clearance are impeded. It is important to tailor suctioning to the irrigation rate during probe activation; otherwise, air can be introduced when aspiration outpaces irrigation inflow, obscuring the field with bubbles. This situation can be avoided by reducing the suction pressure, increasing irrigation height (or pressure), or intermittently clamping the suction tubing to allow enough fluid to remain in the renal pelvis for distension and visualization.[7]

Ureteroscopy: When used in conjunction with a semi-rigid ureteroscope to treat ureteral calculi, a large working channel of at least 5 F is needed to accommodate the smallest probe with an incorporated suction channel (4.5 F). When this is not available, the solid 2.5 F probe is utilized and no suction is possible. Despite these limitations, ureteroscopic success rates between 84% and 100% have been reported.[2]

Disadvantages and Limitations

1. The rigid nature of the ultrasonic probes limits its use in flexible scopes.
2. Technically, when ultrasonic lithotripsy is applied, the stone should be trapped between the probe and the urothelium. Pressure is needed to maintain this relationship, but care should be taken to avoid excessive pressure as perforation is possible, especially in the thin-walled renal pelvis or ureter.
3. Multiple short duration applications of the ultrasonic energy to the stone results in fragmentation. Longer durations of activity provide shorter treatment times but carry the potential to generate a thermal injury and may lead to diminished vision.

References

1. Segura JW, LeRoy AJ. Percutaneous ultrasonic lithotripsy. Urology 1984;23(5 Spec No):7–10.

2. Lasser MS and Pareek G. Percutaneous Lithotripsy and Stone Extraction. Smith's Textbook of Endourology. 3rd edn.

3. Piergiovanni, M., Desgrandchamps, F., Cochand-Priollet,B., et al. Ureteral and bladder lesions after ballistic, ultrasonic, electrohydraulic, or laser lithotripsy. J Endourol1994;8:293–99.

4. Marberger, M. Disintegration of renal and ureteral calculi with ultrasound. Urol Clin North Am 1983;10:729–42.

5. Elder, J.S., Gibbons, R.P., Bush, W.H. Ultrasonic lithotripsy of a large staghorn calculus. J Urol 1984;131:1152–54.

6. Segura, J.W., Patterson, D.E., LeRoy, A.J., et al. Percutaneous removal of kidney stones: review of 1000 cases. J Urol 1985;134:1077–81.

7. Shubha De, Manoj Monga, Bodo E. Knudsen. Basic Energy Modalities in Urologic Surgery. Campbell-Walsh Urology, 9th edn.

PNEUMATIC LITHOTRIPSY

Mechanism of Action

- Pneumatic lithotripsy uses ballistic forces to transfer kinetic energy from a handheld probe to the stone surface. Either compressed gas (medical air or CO_2 cartridges) or electromagnetic oscillations are used to drive a projectile forcefully against the probe tip, thrusting it forward like a piston.[1] Repetitive strikes from the probe tip act as a jackhammer, fragmenting stones at the point of contact. When applied to compliant surfaces such as soft tissue, the impact energy is absorbed and dispersed, whereas rigid objects are not compliant resulting in fracture. Under close visual guidance, the tip of the metal probe is placed into direct contact with the calculus and repetitive impacts result in stone fragmentation.

- Developed in the early 1990s in Switzerland, the Swiss LithoClast uses compressed air to propel a metal projectile against the head of a solid metal probe at a pressure of 3 atmosphere and a rate of 12 Hz.[2] The LithoClast uses medical air and requires a pedal for activation, whereas the lighter weight stone breaker uses a CO_2 cartridge, is triggered by hand, and produces 10 times the impact pressure.

- Successful utilization depends upon the ability to pin a calculus between the urothelium and the tip of the probe. This is understandably more difficult within the confines of the ureter and therefore the utility of pneumatic lithotripsy is best realized during cystolitholapaxy and PCNL, especially during the treatment of large stone burden or exceedingly hard stone compositions.

- Pneumatic lithotripsy is effective in fragmenting harder stones and is less efficient in very soft stones; this is likely because the jackhammer effect produces numerous tiny fragments or because, in the case of extremely soft stones (i.e. matrix stones), the probe punches holes into stones without fragmentation.[1]

Probes

Currently, probes are available in sizes ranging from 0.8 to 2.5 mm and a flexible nickel-titanium (nitinol) probe has been developed to facilitate its use in flexible endoscopy.[3] The development of a suction channel (LithoVac) through which pneumatic lithotripsy is commenced and suction improved the efficiency. The LithoVac is available in several different widths (1.6, 3.5, and 4 mm) (4.8, 10.5 and 12 Fr) and lengths, and facilitates the evacuation of fragments less than 2 mm in size during lithotripsy. Fragments as large as 3.5 mm can be evacuated when the LithoClast is removed from the channel.[4] The application of suction during pneumatic lithotripsy can counteract another major disadvantage of direct contact lithotripsy, retropulsion of stone fragments.[2] In the absence of suction, stone migration occurs in approximately 7.3% of cases.

Tissue Effects

- A survival porcine model was used to test the short-term and long-term effects of 5- to 7-second bursts of LithoClast mucosal exposure to bladder and ureteric urothelium. Histologic changes in immediately sacrificed animals included focal areas of hemorrhage with mucosal erosions and transmural edema. At 3 and 6 weeks, the treated areas were unidentifiable, and histology failed to identify any significant changes.[5]
- In a four-way comparison of intracorporeal lithotripters on iatrogenic urothelial trauma, P Piergiovanni and associates found perpendicular exposure to pneumatic probes to be the least traumatic (compared with laser, ultrasonic lithotripsy, and EHL.[6]

Advantages

- The Clinical Research Office of the Endourological Society reviewed 5800 percutaneous nephrolithotomy procedures (from 96 centers) to assess success rates based on mean Hounsfield units and various surgical characteristics. On regression analysis, pneumatic lithotripsy showed the highest probability of stone-free status (90%) even when compared with combination ultrasonic/pneumatic modalities (82%).[7]
- Other advantages of pneumatic lithotripters are their durability, simplicity of use, and completely reusable components.
- It is the least traumatic to the urothelium as compared to other intracorporeal modalities.[5, 6]
- Adding to dependability are the successful fragmentation of all chemical stone composition[8] and the ability to use interchangeable probes to facilitate stone breakage anywhere in the genitourinary tract.
- Comparing the shearing potential of four intracorporeal lithotripters on endoscopic baskets, pneumatic devices are the only modality not to cut through wire[9]

Disadvantages

- Stone migration is a significant disadvantage when treating ureteric stones because the ballistic effect of the probe can propel stones in capacious ureters into the kidney. Retropulsion has been reported in 10% of distal and 40% of proximal stones treated with pneumatic lithotripsy.
- Ideally, a semirigid ureteroscope with a straight end on working channel should be used for pneumatic stone treatment because bending pneumatic probes reduce the transmitted energy from the generator to the stone.[10] Although 2.4 Fr probes are flexible and can be accommodated by flexible ureteroscopes. An analysis by Zhu[11] quantified the energy loss secondary to probe bending. By measuring tip mechanics, impact momentum decreased 50% and energy by 76% when probe tips were deflected 33°. With 48° of deflection, only 30% of full fragmentation efficiency could be achieved.

References

1. Shubha De, Manoj Monga, Bodo E. Knudsen. Basic Energy Modalities in Urologic Surgery. Campbell-Walsh Urology, 11th edn.

2. Lasser MS and Pareek G. Percutaneous Lithotripsy and Stone Extraction. Smith's Textbook of Endourology. 3rd edn.

3. Tawfiek, E.R., Grasso, M., Bagley, D.H. Initial use of Browne Pneumatic Impactor. J Endourol 1997;11:121–24.

4. Haupt, G., Pannek, J., Herde, T., Schulze, H., Senge, T. The LithoVac: new suction device for the Swiss LithoClast. J Endourol 1995;9:375–57.

5. Denstedt JD, Razvi HA, Rowe E, et al. Investigation of the tissue effects of a new device for intracorporeal lithotripsy—the Swiss LithoClast. J Urol 1995;153:535–37.

6. Piergiovanni, M., Desgrandchamps, F., Cochand-Priollet, B., et al. Ureteral and bladder lesions after ballistic, ultrasonic, electrohydraulic, or laser lithotripsy. J Endourol 1994;8:293–99.

7. Anastasiadis A, Onal B, Modi P, et al. Impact of stone density on outcomes in percutaneous nephrolithotomy (PCNL): an analysis of the

Clinical Research Office of the Endourological Society (CROES) PCNL global study database. Scand J Urol 2013;47:509–14.

8. Teh CL, Zhong P, Preminger GM. Laboratory and clinical assessment of pneumatically driven intracorporeal lithotripsy. J Endourol 1998;12: 163–69.

9. Cordes J, Lange B, Jocham D, et al. Destruction of stone extraction basket during an *in vitro* lithotripsy,

a comparison of four lithotripters. J Endourol 2011;25:1359–62.

10. Grocela, J.A., Dretler, S.P. Intracorporeal lithotripsy. Instrumentation and development. Urol Clin North Am 1997;24:13–23.

11. Zhu S, Kourambas J, Munver R, et al. Quantification of the tip movement of lithotripsy flexible pneumatic probes. J Urol 2000;164:1735–39.

LASER LITHOTRIPSY

Holmium:YAG lasers have revolutionized kidney stone management and flexible ureteroscopy. In conjunction with improved optical systems in actively deflecting ureteroscopes and miniaturized nephroscopes, all areas of the genitourinary tract are now safely accessible for endoscopic lithotripsy using these lasers.[1]

Laser is a mechanism for emitting electromagnetic radiation through stimulated emission of photons. When an atom is stimulated by an external energy source, electrons become metastable and change their orbit. As this excited state decays, an emission of photons (light energy) occurs. There are three differences between laser light and natural light: Laser light is coherent (all photons are in phase), collimated (photons travel parallel to one another), and monochromatic (photons have the same wavelength). It is these characteristics that allow lasers to transmit high energy in a concentrated fashion.[2]

Holmium (Ho): YAG Laser

Mechanism of Action

- The Ho (holmium:yttrium-aluminum-garnet laser) is a solid-state laser operating at a wavelength of 2100 nm. The holmium (Ho):YAG laser is the only laser that is capable of fragmenting all compositions of calculi. It functions through a primary photothermal mechanism that results in stone vaporization.[1, 2] Photothermal fragmentation is accomplished by conversion of light into heat that causes the stone to

melt as well as crack due to the rapidly expanding vapor within the stone.[3] Holmium laser stone fragmentation efficiency increases with increased stone temperature. A "Moses effect" occurs by the rapid vaporization of fluid creating a vapor channel between the fiber tip and stone surface, allowing for more direct energy transfer. This results in the breakdown and disintegration of the heated area, causing craters and fragmentation. As a result of the relatively long pulse rate (250 to 350 μsec), the Ho:YAG laser is considerably less efficient than other shorter pulse lasers. The vapor bubble of the Ho:YAG laser is pear-shaped, leading to increased energy loss laterally, producing weak shock waves with minimal effect on stone fracture.[1]

- The absence of a very strong shock wave minimizes urinary calculus migration away from the laser fiber during lithotripsy, a phenomenon referred to as stone retropulsion. The photothermal effect of the holmium laser contributes to this process via two mechanisms. The first is the creation of a "plume" consisting of vapor bubbles and small stone fragments, which then causes stone migration away from the laser fiber. The second is the generation of internal shock waves within the calculus secondary to the thermal expansion of the water molecules within the stone.[3]

- Although photoacoustic forces are not thought to contribute to fracture, interstitial water vaporization is involved with fragment ejection.

- Laser output can be adjusted based on rate (Hz), energy (J), pulse duration (μsec), and fiber size (μm). The total power output is the product of these two parameters:

$$\text{Total power (W) = Pulse energy (J)} \times \text{Pulse frequency (Hz)}$$

  In the short-pulse mode, the energy delivered by a single laser pulse occurs during a certain period of time (180–330 μs), while in long-pulse mode, the same amount of energy is distributed over a longer period of time (650–1, 215 μs).

- The holmium laser is highly absorbed in water. Given that human tissues are chiefly composed of water, the energy of the Holmium laser is absorbed superficially. As long as the holmium laser laser is fired away from the urothelial mucosa, soft tissue damage is not observed, since the shock wave produced by cavitation bubble collapse is small, and thus much of the photothermal effect of the laser is attenuated by medium between the tip of the laser fiber and the mucosa. In fact, the depth of tissue penetration has previously been proven to be 0.5–1.0 mm.[3–5] This allows for safe use within the collecting system provided that the distance between the tip of the fiber and mucosa is >1 mm.

- Technically, the holmium laser fiber should be kept at least 2 mm beyond the end of the endoscope to avoid damage to the lens system.

- A systematic painting motion represents the ideal use of the holmium laser. This process of lithotripsyallows for vaporization of the stone and avoids the formation of large fragments.

- When performing holmium laser lithotripsy it is important to remain vigilant in monitoring stone position to avoid ureteral injury. Care should be taken not to tunnel through a calculus as perforation through the opposite side may result in urothelial injury.

- Care should be taken to avoid wires, baskets, etc. during laser lithotripsy as the holmium laser is capable of cutting through metal.[6]

Fibers

- The laser energy must be transmitted from the generator to the target. Most commonly silica fibers are used for this purpose, as silica represents a relatively inexpensive, biocompatible means of transmitting Ho: YAG laser energy.[3]

- Holmium laser fibers are available in diameters ranging from 200 to 1000 μm. Both the 200 μm and 365 μm fibers can be used with both semi-rigid and flexible ureteroscopes, and their flexible nature allows for preservation of flexion capabilities during ureteroscopy, a significant advantage.

- Maximal deflection is achieved with 200 μm fibers during flexible ureteroscopy; however, maximal efficiency is seen with 360 μm fibers.

Uses

1. **Ureteroscopy:** Ureteroscopic laser fragmentation can be performed by several techniques.

   Dust-sized fragments are produced by painting the fiber across the surface of a stone. Avoiding the creation of large fragments that are difficult to pass makes basket extraction unnecessary. Using lower energy levels of 0.2 J and higher pulse rates (i.e. 40 Hz) is associated with small debris and minimal retropulsion.

   Increasing pulse energy levels were found to result in larger fragments, with faster fragmentation times. The large pieces can be removed using an endoscopic basket.

   A technique dubbed "popcorning" uses both the photoacoustic and the photothermal mechanisms of laser lithotripsy. Photoacoustic and photothermal properties of a laser are functions of pulse duration and energy. Longer pulse duration produces greater photothermal functionality. Although most Ho:YAG lasers have fixed durations of 250 to 350 μm, adjustable units are becoming more common. Shorter pulses yield higher peak power in resulting shock waves. In a ureteric model, increasing pulse duration from 300 to 700 µm reduced stone retropulsion by 50%.[7] Pulse duration is inversely related to power and can manipulate stone motion depending on the circumstance; this can be helpful in difficult-to-reach anatomy (i.e. lower pole stones) or when numerous fragments exist in a confined area (i.e. minor calyx). The fiber tip is placed several millimeters away from the stones (and mucosa), and shock waves produced by vapor bubbles collapsing cause stones to bounce like popcorn. As stones are agitated, intermittent contact with the laser fiber causes photothermal disintegration. As time passes, the "popcorning" effect continues to produce smaller and smaller fragments, resulting in a fine stone dust, which is passed without consequence. An *in vitro* experiment identified settings of 1.0 J and 20 Hz as giving the most efficient fragmentation when using this technique.[8]

2. Laser fragmentation is central to percutaneous nephrolithotomy performed with reduced diameter sheaths (minipercutaneous, ultra-minipercutaneous, micropercutaneous). Developed initially for pediatrics, the procedure is now used in adults with sheath diameters ranging from 24 Fr (8 mm) to 16 gauge (1.3 mm). Because stone extraction is impossible with extremely narrow sheaths, 200 µm laser fibers are used to dust stones, and debris is cleared by pressurized irrigation or passive urine flow.

Advantages

1. Ability to effectively fragment all stone compositions.
2. The flexible nature of the laser fiber facilitates both flexible ureteroscopy and renoscopy (both antegrade and retrograde).
3. The superficial penetration of the Ho laser provides it with a high margin of safety as long as care is taken to keep the fiber at least 1 mm from the urothelium.

4. In addition, the lack of photoacoustic effects has resulted in the safe use of Ho lithotripsy in patients receiving anticoagulation therapy.[9]

Disadvantages

1. Propensity to perforate the urothelium if activated within close proximity to the wall of the collecting system.
2. The high initial cost of the Ho and its fibers is a deterrent to some institutions.
3. Care should be taken to avoid wires, baskets, etc. during laser lithotripsy as the Ho is capable of cutting through metal.[6]
4. Stone retropulsion is also a concern in laser lithotripsy. In an *in vitro* model the 365 µm and 550 µm fibers were associated with the greatest degree of retropulsion, and the 200 µm fiber with the least.[10]
5. Ho lithotripsy of uric acid stones produces cyanide gas. Despite the theoretical side effects of this, no significant cyanide toxicities have occurred as a result of Ho lithotripsy.[11]

Laser Settings

- Fragment size may be less related to laser lithotripter settings and more dependent on the surgical technique employed, i.e. whether the stone is repeatedly perforated, chipped, or fragmented, in comparison with worked on at the surface, by "dancing" or "painting" it with the laser.[12, 13]
- Lowering the pulse energy or changing to long-pulse mode would decrease the retropulsion effect but would also affect ablation efficiency negatively.
- Pulse energy was the most important factor that determined ablation volume. At the same power levels, low frequency—high pulse energy settings were up to six times more ablative than high frequency—low pulse energy settings.[13, 14] Short-pulse mode is significantly more ablative than the long-pulse mode. The efficiency of the Ho:YAG laser correlates with the pulse energy output, which means higher-power energy

leads to faster fragmentation and shorter operating time.[15]

- Pulse frequency: High pulse frequency (>15 Hz) tends to produce an endoscopic "snowstorm" appearance that requires either increased irrigation pressure or suspension of irradiation until the debris clears for the operator to regain adequate vision.[16] Also, pulse frequencies >10 Hz may be associated with optical fiber tip movement, which causes an increase in the distance between the optical fiber tip and the stone surface, leading to decreased stone irradiation and loss of lithotripsy efficiency.[15, 16]
- Conventionally, energy has been set between 0.5 and 1.0 J and frequency between 5 and 10 Hz.[3, 17, 18] In an *in vitro* study using calyceal calcium oxalate monohydrate stone models, Li and colleagues demonstrated that the fragmentation and vaporization rates associated with the 0.6 J/5 Hz and 0.2 J/50 Hz were comparable.[19]
- Fiber: Larger fibers increase the retropulsion effect when compared to smaller fiber. Larger laser fibers inside narrow working channels also influence irrigation rates negatively, which can impair the surgeons' visualization of structures and, therefore, influence operating time. Larger diameter fibers create wider ablation fissures (p <0.00001), while smaller diameter fibers generate deeper ablation

fissures (p <0.00001), but neither surpassed the other in terms of ablation volume (p = 0.81).[13, 14]

Laser Fiber Degradation

During laser emission, the laser fiber tip degrades because of the "burn-back effect". High pulse energy, small diameter laser fibers, short-pulse mode and harder stones are known to increase the degradation and burn-back of the fiber.[13, 14] Studies have demonstrated that increasing the pulse energy to more than 1 joule will rapidly degrade the small caliber 200 µm fiber.[16]

Suction with Laser

The first reported use of a combination suction and laser device during PCNL comes from Cuellar and Averch.[20] They constructed a hollow, stainless steel tube that could be attached to suction through which they inserted a 365 µm Ho:YAG laser fiber. They report a stone-free rate of 83% in a cohort of 71 patients, with a mean stone size of 3.25 cm suggesting the effectiveness of this novel approach.

Recently several urologic device manufacturers have developed novel instruments, known as laser suction handpieces (LSHP), that couple the Ho:YAG laser with suction for use during PCNL. These include the laser suction tube (Fig. 5.1) (Karl Storz, Germany), LithAssist (Cook Medical), and the suction HP (Lumenis, Israel) with outer diameters of the

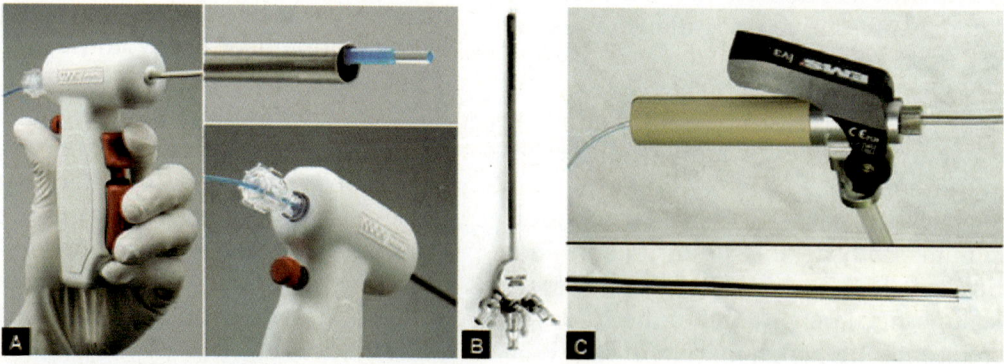

Fig. 5.1: Laser suction handpieces: (A) LithAssist (Cook Medical); (B) Laser suction tube (Storz); (C) Suction with laser sheath for MiniPERC (EMS)

suction tubes of 12 F, 11.6 F, and 11.3 F respectively.[21, 22] Due to the small luminal size and limited suction, low pulse energy, high frequency laser settings, commonly referred to as dusting are advisable in an effort to reduce stone into a fine powder amenable to evacuation.[22]

A 4.5 Fr suction tube with a laser sheath for a 365 µm fiber has been introduced by EMS. This can pass through the working channels of the miniaturized PCNL scopes.[23]

References

1. Shubha De, Manoj Monga, Bodo E. Knudsen. Basic Energy Modalities in Urologic Surgery. Campbell-Walsh Urology, 11th edn.

2. Lasser MS and Pareek G. Percutaneous Lithotripsy and Stone Extraction. Smith's Textbook of Endourology. 3rd edn.

3. Pierre S, Preminger GM. Holmium laser for stone management. World J Urol 2007;25:235–39.

4. Santa-Cruz, R.W., Leveillee, R.J., Krongrad, A. *Ex vivo* comparison of four lithotripters commonly used in the ureter: What does it take to perforate? J Endourol 1998;12:417–22.

5. Wollin, T.A., Denstedt, J.D. The holmium laser in urology. J Clin Laser Med Surg 1998;16:13–20.

6. Freiha, G.S., Glickman, R.D., Teichman, J.M. Holmium:YAG laser-induced damage to guide-wires: experimental study. J Endourol 1997;11: 331–36.

7. Finley DS, Petersen J, Abdelshehid C, et al. Effect of holmium:YAG laser pulse width on lithotripsy retropulsion *in vitro*. J Endourol 2005;19:1041–44.

8. Chawla SN, Chang MF, Chang A, et al. Effectiveness of high-frequency holmium:YAG laser stone fragmentation: the "popcorn effect." J Endourol 2008;22:645 50.

9. Kuo, R.L., Aslan, P., Fitzgerald, K.B., Preminger, G.M. Use of ureteroscopy and holmium: YAG laser in patients with bleeding diatheses. Urology 1998;52:609–13.

10. White, M.D., Moran, M.E., Calvano, C.J., Borhan-Manesh, A., Mehihaff, B.A. Evaluation of retropulsion caused by holmium:YAG laser with various power settings and fibers. J Endourol 1998;12:183–86.

11. Teichman, J.M., Vassar, G.J., Glickman, R.D., Beserra, C.M.,Cina, S.J., Thompson, I.M. Holmium:YAG lithotripsy: photothermal mechanism converts uric acid calculi to cyanide. J Urol 1998; 160:320–24.

12. Teichman JM, Bellman GC, et al. Holmium:YAG lithotripsy yields smaller fragments than lithoClast, pulsed dye laser or electrohydraulic lithotripsy. J. Urol 1998;159(1):17–23.

13. Kronenberg P, Traxer O. *In vitro* fragmentation efficiency of holmium:yttrium-aluminum-garnet (YAG) laser lithotripsy: a comprehensive study encompassing different frequencies, pulse energies, total power levels and laser fiber diameters. BJU Int 2014;114(2):261–67.

14. Traxer O, Kronenberg P. Update on lasers in urology 2014: current assessment on holmium: yttrium-aluminum-garnet (Ho:YAG) laser lithotripter settings and laser fibers. World J Urol 2015;33: 463.

15. Sun Y, Gao X, et al. 70 W Holmium:Yttrium-Aluminum-Garnet Laser in Percutaneous Nephrolithotomy for Staghorn Calculi. J Endourol 2009; 23:1687–91.

16. Spore SS, Teichman JMH, et al. Holmium:YAG Lithotripsy: Optimal Power Settings. J Endourol 1999;13:559–66.

17. Glickman L, Munver R. Comparison of low power/high frequency holmium laser settings with conventional settings on ureteral and renal stone fragmentation efficiency. J Urol 2015;193:e888–89.

18. Sea J, Jonat LM, Chew BH, et al. Optimal power settings for Holmium:YAG lithotripsy. J Urol 2012;187:914–19.

19. Li R, Ruckle D, et al. High Frequency Dusting Versus Conventional Holmium Laser Lithotripsy for Intrarenal and Ureteral Calculi. J Endourol 2017;31:272–77.

20. Cuellar DC, Averch TD. Holmium laser percutaneous nephrolithotomy using a unique suction device. J Endourol 2004;18:780–82.

21. Okhunov Z, del Junco M, Yoon R, et al. *In vitro* evaluation of LithAssist. A novel combined holmium laser and suction device. J Endourol 2014;28:980–84.

22. Dauw CA., Borofsky MS., York N and Lingeman JE. A Usability Comparison of Laser Suction Handpieces for Percutaneous Nephrolithotomy. J Endourology 2016;30:1165–68.

23. Laser with Suction as an Energy Source in Mini Percutaneous Nephrolithotomy: Muljibhai Patel Urological Hospital Experience. Singh A, Jairath A, et al. J Endourol. Videourology. Oct 2016.

DUAL MODALITY LITHOTRIPTERS

Ultrasonic lithotripters, although relatively inefficient at fragmenting hard stones, provide the advantage of concurrent suction, often eliminating the need for manual endoscopic extraction. Conversely, pneumatic lithotripters, which are not typically equipped with suction control, have proven superior at fragmenting stones of all consistencies. However, subsequent retrieval of fragments can prove to be both tedious and time-consuming.[1, 2]

Newer modalities have been developed by combining ultrasonic and pneumatic lithotripters into a single handpiece. Olbert and colleagues were one of the first to describe the efficacy of combined ultrasonic and pneumatic lithotripsy probes when they published their experience with the LithoClast Master in 2003.[3] This device was tested against ultrasonic and pneumatic systems and was found to provide superior stone fragmentation rates. The Swiss LithoClast Ultra, CyberWand (Olympus) and shock pulse (olympus). Figure 5.3 use different strategies to capitalize on the advantages of each modality. Pneumatic lithotripsy is effective at fragmenting harder stones, whereas ultrasonic action produces smaller fragments, while simultaneously removing them from the field. These hybrid systems are available only as rigid probes and can be used only in transurethral or percutaneous procedures.[1]

LithoClast Ultra

The LithoClast Ultra was the first dual modality lithotripter, combining two independently functioning handpieces that are fixed together. The front piece houses the ultrasonic lithotripter, with a central channel allowing throughway for the slender pneumatic probe (Fig. 5.2). The 1 mm solid pneumatic probe sits within the suction channel of the 3.3 or 3.8 mm hollow ultrasonic probe (Fig. 5.4). The pneumatic frequency can be adjusted from 2 to 12 Hz, and function in single or continuous

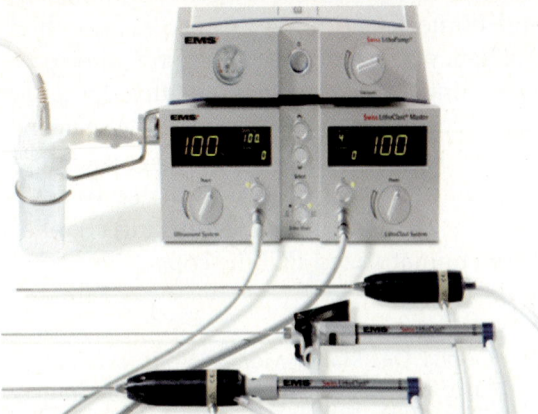

Fig. 5.2: Dual modality lithotripters: LithoClast Ultra

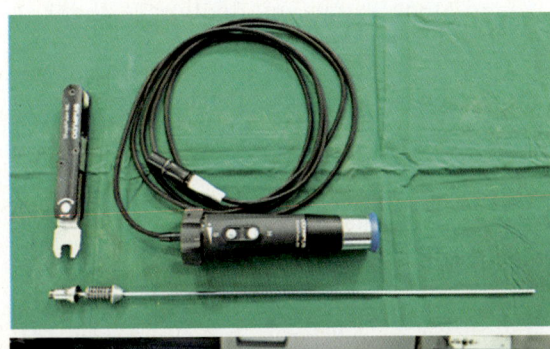

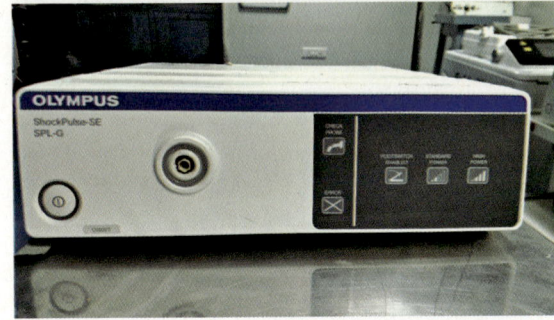

Fig. 5.3: Dual modality lithotripters: Shock Pulse

pulse modes. The ultrasound component allows adjustment of the duty and power, with a frequency of 24 to 26 kHz.[4] A composite pedal allows selective or combined use of each modality. Three cords attach to the handpiece for medical air, ultrasonic power, and suction. In-line suction allows continuous fragment removal and collection (using a stone trap) and handpiece cooling. For maximal control,

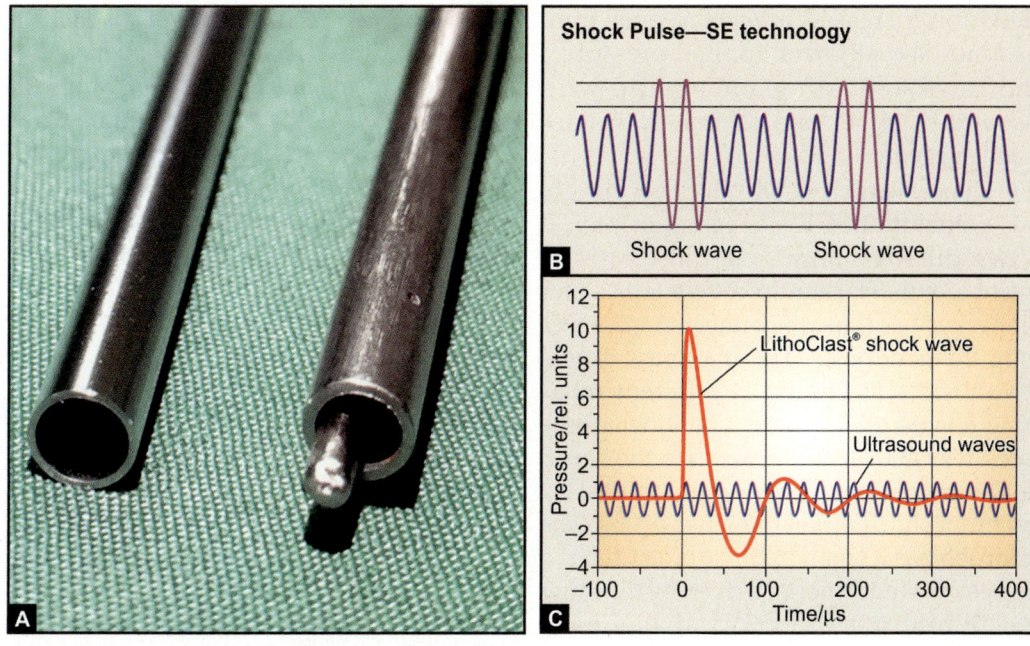

Fig. 5.4A to C: Comparison of the LithoClast Ultra vs the Shock Pulse. (A) Shock Pulse: 3.76 mm single probe with 3.2 mm suction channel; LithoClast Ultra: 3.8 mm ultrasound probe with 1 mm pneumatic probe within with reduced suction channel; (B) Shock Pulse: Constant ultrasonic wave energy with intermittent electrokinetic or ballistic shock wave energy at a high rate of recurrence (300 Hz); (C) LithoClast Ultra: Choice of activating pneumatic with ultrasound or either one separately resides with the surgeon

the tip of the pneumatic probe should be slightly recessed from the outer ultrasonic probe. In this way, the ultrasonic probe can make maximal contact with the stone surface, and pneumatic retropulsion is limited. When activated, the pneumatic tip advances and strikes the stone beyond the ultrasonic probe tip. If large immobile stones are being treated (i.e. staghorn calculi), better fragmentation can be achieved by adjusting the pneumatic probe 2.5 mm past the ultrasonic sheath; however, simultaneous treatment of smaller fragments may become more challenging. In a prospective randomized comparison, Lehman and associates randomized 30 patients needing PCNL to either combination pneumatic and ultrasonic lithotripsy or standard ultrasonic lithotripsy.[5] Stone location and burden were similar in both groups, and all procedures were performed successfully. When classified by stone type, the combination unit was faster for fragmentation in the hard stone group (calcium oxalate monohydrate, cystine, or calcium phosphate), but slower in the soft stone group. There was no difference identified in stone retrieval times, mean operative time, mechanical failure rate, or mean estimated blood loss. Stone penetration time improved when either pneumatic frequency or ultrasonic power was increased.[6] The quickest time was obtained with pneumatic settings of 12 Hz and 100% ultrasonic power. In this study, pneumatic frequency accounted for 79% of the overall effect. Goldmann and coworkers[7] evaluated the effect of probe pressure and rotation on LithoClast Master efficiency. The ultrasound only component functioned best at 1000 g pressure and 90° of rotation. Combination ultrasonic and pneumatic was affected by pressure, rotation, and pneumatic frequency. The 1000 g pressure was shown most effective, and higher pneumatic settings again functioned better. Overall, they showed the combination increased efficiency over pure ultrasound only at lower applied pressure.

Choice of activating pneumatic with ultrasound or either one separately resides with the surgeon.

The CyberWand (ACMI, Southborough, MA) is a dual probe ultrasonic lithotripter. It uses two different ultrasonic pulse rates to fragment calculi. The handpiece contains outer and inner probes that are connected via a free mass in the handpiece. The free mass causes the two probes to vibrate at different rates, creating a synergistic effect. The inner probe vibrates at 21,000 Hz and is fixed to the handpiece. The outer probe vibrates closer to 1000 Hz and is 1 mm shorter than the inner probe. The outer probe has a small ballistic effect related to the free mass and energy driven by the inner probe. While the CyberWand has been demonstrated to be an effective lithotripter, concern has been raised regarding the noise generated during its use compared with other lithotripters.[8] If used for more than 90 minutes per day, only the CyberWand is above the threshold set by the U.S. Department of Labor and Occupational Health and Safety Administration for risk of noise-related occupational hearing loss.

The Shock Pulse (Olympus) offers a large single lumen probe that delivers constant ultrasonic wave energy with intermittent electrokinetic or ballistic shock wave energy at a high rate of recurrence (300 Hz). It offers the advantage of a larger inner lumen for simultaneous removal of fragments.

The Shock Pulse intracorporeal lithotripter consists of a handpiece transducer, which houses piezoelectric elements that produce 21,000 Hz of ultrasonic energy. The handpiece also contains a suction control dial, allowing for hand activated suction control (Fig. 5.3). The single-probe design employs free mass elements at the proximal end of the probe, which oscillate to produce mechanical shock waves. These shock waves are transmitted to an adjacent return spring, which then propagate down the probe, delivering 300 Hz of mechanical energy. The 3.76 mm Shock Pulse probe has the largest suction lumen of any existing device, measuring 3.2 mm (Fig. 5.4). Based on the results of *in vitro* experiments, Chew BH and colleagues concluded that the Shock Pulse system is equally as effective as the other dual modality lithotripters and in some regards, perhaps even more effective.[2]

References

1. Shubha De, Manoj Monga, Bodo E. Knudsen. Basic Energy Modalities in Urologic Surgery. Campbell-Walsh Urology, 11th edn.

2. Chew BN, Matteliano AA, et al. Benchtop and Initial Clinical Evaluation of the Shock Pulse Stone Eliminator in Percutaneous Nephrolithotomy. J Endourol 2017;31:191–97.

3. Olbert P, Weber J, Hegel A, et al. Combining LithoClast and ultrasound power in one device for percutaneous nephrolithotomy: *In vitro* results of a novel and highly effective technology. Urology 2003;61:55–59.

4. Lowe G, Knudsen BE. Ultrasonic, Pneumatic and Combination Intracorporeal Lithotripsy for Percutaneous Nephrolithotomy. J Endourol 2009;23:1663–68.

5. Lehman DS, Hruby GW, Phillips C, Venkatesh R, Best S, Monga M, Landman J. Prospective randomized comparison of a combined ultrasonic and pneumatic lithotrite with a standard ultrasonic lithotrite for percutaneous nephrolithotomy. J Endourol 2008;22:285–89.

6. Kuo RL, Paterson RF, Siqueira TM Jr, Evan AP, McAteer JA, Williams JC Jr, Lingeman JE. *In vitro* assessment of LithoClast Ultra intracorporeal lithotripter. J Endourol 2004;18: 153–56. Soucy F, Ko R, Denstedt JD, Razvi H. Occupational noise exposure during endourologic procedures. J Endourol 2008;22:1609–11.

7. Goldman DM, Pedro RN, Kossett A, Durfee W, Monga M. Maximizing stone fragmentation efficiency with ultrasonic probes: Impact of probe pressure and rotation. J Urol 2009;181:1429–33.

8. Soucy F, Ko R, Denstedt JD, Razvi H. Occupational noise exposure during endourologic procedures. J Endourol 2008;22:1609–11.

Rajesh Kukreja

6 | Exit Strategy Post-PCNL

After completion of stone removal, traditionally a nephrostomy tube has been inserted with the intention to both drain the urine and tamponade the access tract, establishing hemostasis. Other possible benefits of the nephrostomy tube are clearance of blood, avoiding clots, prevent urinary extravasation, drain purulent fluid, maintenance of the re-entry tract for a staged procedure and contrast study in the postoperative period.

There are a variety of choices for the nephrostomy tubes.[1]

1. **The Foley and Councill catheters** used for transurethral drainage can be used as nephrostomy tubes as well. Typically 16 to 24 Fr catheters are used for postoperative nephrostomy drainage. The 5 ml retention balloon might be too large for some collecting systems and does not need to be completely inflated. The balloon can cause calyceal obstruction if it is pulled into an infundibulum. Saline or water should be used to inflate the balloon because viscous contrast material might hinder emptying of the balloon when removal is attempted. An advantage of the Councill catheter is the ability to pass a small-caliber catheter through the end hole and down the ureter, providing more secure access to the upper urinary tract collecting system and maintaining ureteral patency. All nephrostomy tubes, even ones with robust internal retention devices, should be fixed to the skin externally with a suture or other mechanism.

2. **Malecot catheter:** This provides a non-obstructive retention mechanism. The Malecot catheter is also available with an extension that is directed down the ureter. This modification is called a "re-entry" catheter, because it simplifies placing a guidewire through the Malecot catheter and down the ureter into the bladder. The extension is long enough (18 cm) so that in most patients the Malecot tube can be withdrawn until the wings are externalized and a guidewire can be placed into the ureter. Malecot catheters for renal use are large-bore catheters, ranging from 12 to 30 Fr.

3. **Cope catheter:** Cope nephrostomy tubes provide a more secure retention mechanism. A string exits the catheter a few centimeters from the distal tip and then re-enters the catheter near the tip. Pulling on the string forms a secure coil that is not easily dislodged from the renal pelvis. They are available in sizes ranging from 6 to 14 Fr. The Cope retention mechanism is also used in nephroureteral stents. A nephroureteral stent has a renal coil-like that of a Cope nephrostomy tube, but the tube continues onto a ureteral extension that travels down the ureter to end in a passive pigtail that

rests in the bladder. A nephroureteral stent offers excellent control of the entire upper urinary tract, from renal pelvis to bladder, and is unlikely to become dislodged. Nephroureteral stents are available in diameters of 8.5 or 10.2 Fr, and the standard lengths (from renal to bladder coil) are 20 to 28 cm.

4. Abdominal drainage tubes with multiple holes at the distal end offer excellent drainage but need to be fixed securely as they do not have any self-retaining mechanism. Specially designed tube catheters with radiopaque tips to allow proper positioning of the tip in the pelvicalyceal system are available in varying sizes. An 8 or 10 Fr infant feeding tube can be used and passed over the wire into the ureter to allow secured positioning.

All these types of nephrostomy tubes can be passed over a guidewire and allow re-entry mechanism. The potential for tube dislodgement favors nephrostomy tubes with self-retaining mechanisms or those with some extension down the ureter to maintain a conduit to the upper urinary tract collecting system, even if the renal pelvic portion of the tube is pulled out of the kidney.

Tubeless PCNL

The possible disadvantages of nephrostomy tube placement have been patient discomfort and pain. The nephrostomy tube matures the tract and establishes an anomalous path for urinary leakage post-tube removal leading to increased morbidity and prolonged hospitalization. Therefore, the practice of routine placement of nephrostomy tube after an uncomplicated PCNL with complete calculus clearance has been questioned.

- From initial reports by Wickham and associates in 1984[2] and Bellman and coworkers[3] in 1997 to the several series recently published, the tubeless percutaneous nephrolithotomy (PCNL) has been repeatedly tested and proven.[4–10]

- A significant reduction in pain scores was seen by replacing the standard large bore (>20 Fr) nephrostomy draining tube by a small bore (10 Fr) tube. Randomised comparative studies by Desai,[11] Feng[12] and their colleagues revealed least amount of narcotic requirement, the shortest hospital stay, and the shortest duration of percutaneous tract site urine leak in the tubeless group as compared to the large-bore and small-bore nephrostomy drainage tube groups. In the study by Desai and colleagues,[11] none of the patients showed evidence of perinephric urinary collection on postoperative renal ultrasonography. There were no read missions to the hospital and no patient required any ancillary procedures.

- Borges and colleagues did a systematic review and meta-analysis of 10 randomized comparative trials of nephrostomy placement versus tubeless PCNL.[13] The meta-analysis highlights were:
  a. Hemoglobin drop: No difference between the tubeless PCNL and conventional PCNL.
  b. Prolonged urine drainage was reported as a complication in three studies. The incidence was lower in the tubeless group than in the conventional group.
  c. Reduced postoperative pain
  d. There was no difference between the groups concerning postoperative fever.
  e. A benefit of shorter length of hospital stay in the tubeless PCNL group.

- Results from The Global PCNL Study from The Clinical Research Office Endourology Society suggests that tubeless percutaneous nephrolithotomy leads to shorter hospital stay and reduced postoperative pain in comparison to use of large post-procedure nephrostomy tubes, but that these benefits are less certain in comparison to small nephrostomy tubes.[14]

- The tubeless approach appears to be safe even when supracostal access is used and in the setting of bilateral simultaneous procedures.[15–17]

Ureteral Drainage in Tubeless PCNL

Options for ureteral stenting without a nephrostomy tube after percutaneous renal surgery include an internal ureteral stent that is removed cystoscopically, an internal ureteral stent with an attached string that exits out of the flank to allow removal of the ureteral stent without cystoscopy, and an externalized (out the urethra) ureteral stent that is removed along with the urethral catheter to which it is attached.[1]

Majority of the tubeless study patients had a double J stent placed to promote urinary flow down the ureters as was evident in 8 of the 10 RCTs assessed by Borges et al.[13] This is associated with potential for stent dysuria and the need for an additional procedure for stent removal. Shah and colleagues found that 30% of the patients experienced discomfort related to double-J placement.[15] Similarly, 52.1% of the patients had some sort of stent-related symptom in a study by Gonen and colleagues.[18] A randomized prospective study using a validated QoL assessment instrument specific for nephrolithiasis by Zhao and group showed that QoL is significantly worse with tubeless patients with double-J stent placement than with temporary nephrostomy drainage in the immediate aftermath following PCNL.[19]

Goh and Wolf first reported the use of an externalized ureteral stent (single pigtail) as an alternative to a postoperative nephrostomy tube.[4]

Lojanapiwat and colleagues in 2001 used 6 Fr ureteral catheter as an external stent for 48 hours following a tubeless PCNL and demonstrated reduced postoperative morbidity without increasing complications.[20] Gonen and colleagues reported that using an EUC instead of a double-J (DJ) stent for postoperative drainage did not increase postoperative morbidity of the tubeless PCNL.[18] Similarly, Mouracade and colleagues concluded that replacement of DJ with EUC in tubeless PCNL was a safe and effective procedure for patients with a mean stone burden of 17.25 mm.[21] Zhou and colleagues in a randomized prospective study compared the outcomes following use of externalized ureteral catheter (EUC) vs double-J (DJ) ureteral stent in tubeless minimally invasive percutaneous nephrolithotomy (MPCNL).[22] There were no statistically significant differences between the two groups regarding the mean operative times, mean VAS scores, analgesic requirements, mean hemoglobin drop, mean hospital stay, and overall complication rate. However, compared with DJ group, EUC group presented fewer postoperative stent-related symptoms and less occurrence of severe VUR ($p < 0.05$). Patients with pyuria, perforation of the renal collecting system, severe intraoperative or postoperative hemorrhage, second-look procedure necessity and presence of residual calculi >4 mm were excluded from the study.

The advent of miniaturised PCNL has led to an increased incidence of tubeless procedures due to the reduced bleeding. In a series of 94 patients treated with Ultra-miniPERC (UMP) for stones ranging from 1 to 2 cm, 92% were tubeless.[23] Similar results were noted by Mishra[24] and Knoll[25] in their series as well. Tubeless procedures directly impacts length of stay, postoperative pain and ultimately patient satisfaction. Most patients who undergo UMP have a ureteral catheter but this is removed at 12 to 24 hours, thus, overcoming the need of an indwelling double-J stent.[23] Stents result in symptoms, health care cost, decreased quality of life and further procedure to facilitate removal. In another series of 318 miniPERCs, the VAS at 48 hours was minimum in patients with tubeless procedure with ureteral catheter drainage. It was intermediate in patients with nephrostomy drainage, and maximum inpatients with the DJ stent drainage group.[26]

Totally Tubeless PCNL

More recently, the concept of a "totally tubeless" percutaneous renal surgery, omitting both the nephrostomy tube and ureteral catheter, has been introduced. This can be considered in selected patients with low-volume stones, a traumatic single access, and no hemorrhage, perforation, or obstruction. A meta-analysis of five randomized controlled trials and four non-randomized comparative studies comparing "totally tubeless" percutaneous nephrolithotomy to percutaneous nephrolithotomy with a post-procedure nephrostomy tube suggests that the "totally tubeless" approach reduces hospital stay, analgesic requirement, and time to return to normal activity without increasing complications.[27]

Adjuncts to Tubeless PCNL

Several authors tried to use sealant agents in the percutaneous tract to improve hemostasis.[28–32] In an RCT, Singh and associates studied the absorbable gelatin Spongostan. No benefits could be observed for the gelatin-group. In a similar manner, fibrin sealant and Surgicel also failed to improve the outcomes of tubeless PCNL. Aron and colleagues retrospectively studied direct diathermal coagulation of bleeding vessels, and no hemostatic benefit was reported. On the other hand, Jou and coworkers published a reduction in the blood transfusion rate when electrocauterization was applied. Overall, the usefulness of any of the adjuncts for tract hemostasis is not certain and further studies are necessary.

In a randomized controlled trial, Shah and colleagues demonstrated that nephrostomy tract infiltration of bupivacaine in tubeless PCNL is associated with less postoperative pain and analgesia requirement.[33] 74.6% of these patients had a supracostal access. Local infiltration of the nephrostomy tract, including the renal capsule, was performed under fluoroscopy guidance in patients undergoing tubeless PCNL. Because this was performed with the Amplatz sheath in place, the authors believe that the local anesthetic drug would have had its effect even on the renal capsule and deeper muscle layers. Dalela and coworkers[34] had emphasized that "most of the pain at the time of PCNL is experienced during dilatation of the renal capsule and the parenchyma as it is richly innervated by pain conducting neurons." They presented a series of PCNL performed using their technique of local anesthesia that included a renal capsular block. Adapting a similar hypothesis, Jonnavithula and colleagues[35] infiltrated 20 ml of 0.25% bupivacaine, under fluoroscopy guidance, with a 23-gauge spinal needle (10 cm length) along the nephrostomy tube at 6 o'clock and 12 o'clock positions (10 ml in each tract), including renal capsule, muscles, subcutaneous tissue, and skin. It was their assumption that all these structures contribute to development of postoperative pain. In a randomized controlled study, they found their technique to be associated with significant reduction in pain scores and analgesic requirement without any complications.

CONCLUSION

The practice of nephrostomy tube omission with an external ureteral catheter drainage for 24–48 hours avoids many of the disadvantages of a nephrostomy tube and an internal ureteral stent but still leaves the problem of loss of access in case a secondary procedure is required. With improved endoscopes, better ancillary tools, and growing experience with percutaneous surgery, the need for secondary procedures is declining. In properly selected patients including those who do not for some other reason need external drainage (e.g. pyonephrosis, significant bleeding, significant collecting system injury) and those who are unlikely to need a secondary procedure, omission of the postoperative nephrostomy tube appears to be safe and effective.

References

1. J Stuart Wolf. Percutaneous Approaches to the Upper UrinaryTract Collecting System. Campbell-Walsh Urology, 11th edition.

2. Wickham JE, Miller RA, Kellett MJ, Payne SR. Percutaneous nephrostolithotomy: One stage or two? Br J Urol 1984;56:582–85.

3. Bellman GC, Davidoff R, Candela J, Gerspach J, Kurtz S, Stout L. Tubeless percutaneous renal surgery. J Urol 1997;157:1578–82.

4. Goh, M., Wolf, J. S., Jr: Almost totally tubeless percutaneous nephrolithotomy: further evaluation of the technique. J Endourol 1999;13:177.

5. Limb, J., Bellman, G. C.: Tubeless percutaneous renal surgery:review of first 112 patients. Urology 2002;59–527.

6. Pietrow PK, Auge BK, Lallas CD, Santa-Cruz RW, Newman GE, Albala DM, Preminger GM. Pain after percutaneous nephrolithotomy: Impact of nephrostomy tube size. J Endourol 2003;17:411–14.

7. Maheshwari PN, Andankar MG, Bansal M. Nephrostomy tube after percutaneous nephrolithotomy: Large-bore versus pigtail catheter? J Endourol 2000;14:735–38.

8. Gupta NP, Kesarwani P, Goel R, Aron M. Tubeless percutaneous nephrolithotomy. A comparative study with standard percutaneous nephrolithotomy. Urol Int 2005;74:58–61.

9. Agrawal MS, Agrawal M, Gupta A, et al. A randomized comparison of tubeless and standard percutaneous nephrolithotomy. J Endourol 2008;22:439–42.

10. Shah HN, Sodha HS, Khandkar AA, et al. A randomized trial evaluating type of nephrostomy drainage after percutaneous nephrolithotomy: Small bore vs tubeless. J Endourol 2008;22:1433–39.

11. Desai MR, Kukreja RA, Desai MM, Mhaskar SS, Wani KA,Patel SH, Bapat SD. A prospective randomized comparison of type of nephrostomy drainage following percutaneous nephrostolithotomy: Large bore versus small bore versus tubeless. J Urol 2004;172:565–67.

12. Feng MI, Tamaddon K, Mikhail A, Kaptein JS, Bellman GC. Prospective randomized study of various techniques of percutaneous nephrolithotomy. Urology 2001;58:345–50.

13. Borges CF, Fregonesi A, et al. Systematic review and meta-analysis of 10 randomized comparative

trials of nephrostomy placement versus tubeless PCNL. J Endourol 2010;24:1739–46.

14. Cormio L, Gonzalez GI, Tolley D, et al. Exit strategies following percutaneous nephrolithotomy (PCNL): a comparison of surgical outcomes in the Clinical Research Office of the Endourological Society (CROES) PCNL Global Study. World J Urol 2013; 31:1239–44.

15. Shah HN, Kausik VB, Hegde SS, Shah JN, Bansal MB.Tubeless percutaneous nephrolithotomy:A prospective feasibility study and review of previous reports. BJU Int 2005;96:879–83.

16. Duty B, Conlin M, Wagner M, et al. Supracostal tubeless percutaneous nephrolithotomy: a retrospective cohort study. J Endourol 2013;27:294–97.

17. Jun-Ou J, Lojanapiwat B. Supracostal access: does it affect tubeless percutaneous nephrolithotomy efficacy and safety? Int Braz J Urol 2010;36:171–76.

18. Gonen M, Ozturk B, Ozkardes H. Double-J stenting compared with one night externalized ureteral catheter placement in tubeless percutaneous nephrolithotomy. J Endourol 2009;23:27–32.

19. Zhao PT, Hoenig DM, Smith AD, et al. A Randomized Controlled Comparison of Nephrostomy Drainage vs Ureteral Stent Following Percutaneous Nephrolithotomy Using the Wiscons in Stone QoL. J Endourol 2016;30:1275–84.

20. Lojanapiwat B, Soonthornphan S, Wudhikarn S. Tubeless percutaneous nephrolithotomy in selected patients. J Endourol 2001;15:711–13.

21. Mouracade P, Spie R, Lang H, Jacqmin D, Saussine C. Tubeless percutaneous nephrolithotomy: What about replacing the Double-J stent with a ureteral catheter. J Endourol 2008;22:273–75.

22. Zhou Y, Zhu J, et al. Randomized Study of Ureteral Catheter vs Double-J Stent in Tubeless Minimally Invasive Percutaneous Nephrolithotomy Patients. J Endourol 2017;31:278–82.

23. Desai J, et al. Prospective Outcomes of Ultra-mini Percutaneous Nephrolithotomy: A Consecutive Cohort Study. J Urol 2016;195:741–46.

24. Mishra S, Sharma R, et al. Prospective comparative study of MiniPERC and standard PNL for treatment of 1 to 2 cm size renal stone. BJUI 2011;108:896–900.

25. Knoll T, Wezel F, Michel MS, et al. Do Patients Benefit from Miniaturized Tubeless Percutaneous

Nephrolithotomy? A Comparative Prospective Study. J Endourol 2010 24(7):1075–9.

26. Bhattu AS, Mishra S, Ganpule A, et al. Outcomes in a Large Series of MiniPERCs: Analysis of Consecutive 318 Patients. J Endourol 2015; 29(3): 283–87.

27. Zhong Q, Zheng C, Mo J, et al. Total tubeless versus standard percutaneous nephrolithotomy: a meta-analysis. J Endourol 2013;27:420–26.

28. Singh I, Saran RN, Jain M. Does sealing of the tract with absorbable gelatin (Spongostan), facilitate tubeless PCNL? A prospective study. J Endourol 2008;22:2485–93.

29. Shah HN, Hedge S, Shah JN, et al. A prospective randomized trial evaluating the safety and efficacy of fibrin sealantin tubeless percutaneous nephrolithotomy. J Urol 2006;176:2488–93.

30. Aghamir SM, Khazaeli MH, Meisami A. Use of Surgicel for sealing nephrostomy tract after totally tubeless percutaneous nephrolithotomy. J Endourol 2006;20:293–95.

31. Aron M, Goel R, Kesarwani PK, Gupta NP. Hemostasis in tubeless PNL: Point of technique. Urol Int 2004;73:244–47.

32. Jou YC, Cheng MC, Sheen JH, et al. Electro-cauterization of bleeding points for percuta-neous nephrolithotomy. Urology 2004;64: 443–47.

33. Shah HN, Shah RH, et al. A Randomized Control Trial Evaluating Efficacy of Nephrostomy Tract Infiltration with Bupivacaine after Tubeless Percutaneous Nephrolithotomy. J Endourol 2012;26:478–83.

34. Dalela D, Goel A, Singh P, Shankhwar SN. Renal capsular block: A novel method for performing percutaneous nephrolithotomy under local anesthesia. J Endourol 2004;18:544–46.

35. Jonnavithula N, Pisapati MV, Durga P, et al. Efficacy of peritubal local anesthetic infiltration in alleviating postoperative pain in percuta-neous nephrolithotomy. J Endourol 2009;23: 857–60.

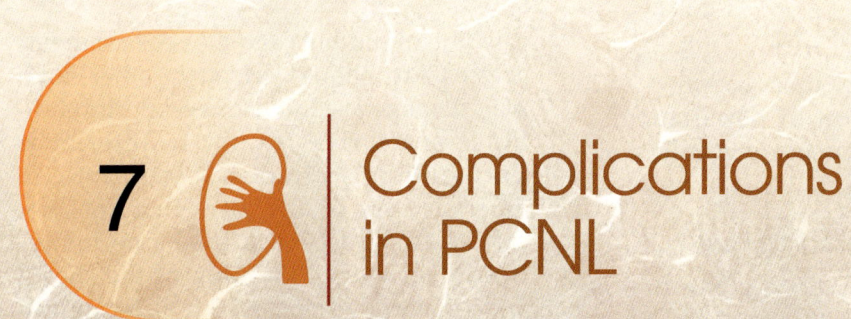

7 Complications in PCNL

Rajesh Kukreja

Despite the fact that percutaneous renal surgery is associated with lower morbidity, it is not without its share of complications. Lang performed a large multi-institutional survey of patients undergoing PCNL. The overall complication rate was reported to be 26%.[1] The complication rates had a direct correlation with experience and decreased from 61% to 3.7% with an increase in the level of experience.[2]

Complications are generally related to the initial puncture with injury of renal blood vessels and the surrounding organs (e.g. pleura, colon, spleen, liver, lung). The most common complications include postoperative bleeding and fever. The severity of complications has been categorized using the Dindo-modified Clavien system[3] (Table 7.1). Major complications (Clavien grade 3 or greater) occur in 4–5% of the patients[3,4] (Table 7.2).

Table 7.1: Clavien system of grading of complications	
Grade	Description
0	No complication
I	Deviation from the normal postoperative course without the need for intervention
II	Minor complications requiring pharmacological intervention, including blood transfusion and total parenteral nutrition
IIIa	Complications requiring surgical, endoscopic or radiological intervention, but self-limited, without general anesthesia
IIIb	Complications requiring surgical, endoscopic radiological intervention, but self-limited, with general anesthesia
IVa	Life-threatening complications requiring intensive care unit management; single organ dysfunction, including dialysis
IVb	Life-threatening complications requiring intensive care unit management; multi-organ dysfunction
V	Death resulting from complications

Table 7.2: Clavien complications in percutaneous surgery							
	N	Clavien grade (%)					
		0	1	2	3	4	5
Seitz et al	11929	77	11	7	4.1	0.6	0.04
Labate et al	5724	79	16			4.2	

HAEMORRHAGE: POST-PCNL

Acute hemorrhage is the most common and significant complication of percutaneous access into the upper urinary tract collecting system.[5]

Pathophysiology of Bleeding Post-PCNL

- A key requisite to stone clearance is establishing optimal access to the renal collecting system. A high-flow arterio-venous network constituting 20% of the total cardiac output closely surrounds the collecting system. Most hemorrhage occurs from the renal parenchyma, and in most cases this hemorrhage is not significant. Small arteries and veins are always injured to some degree by percutaneous entry into the kidney. Parenchymal bleeding is minimized by proper entry and dilation and by careful manipulation of the sheath, but it still can occur[5] (Table 7.3).

- Significant vessels are the segmental and the interlobar vessels. Access to the pelvicalyceal system and intrarenal manipulations may traumatize these vessels, resulting in significant bleeding. Excessive bleeding can occur during needle passage, tract dilatation, and during nephroscopy or in the postoperative period.[6–9]

- Being a minimally invasive modality, direct control of bleeding through the PCNL tracts is generally not possible. The mainstay of reducing bleeding is meticulous operative technique with identification and possible modification of factors that may increase or decrease bleeding.

- An ideal puncture should be straight, traversing the shortest distance from the skin to the target calyx and aligned with the infundibulum and the renal pelvis in a straight line. This would transverse the minimum distance through the cortex and potentially avoids the larger renal vessels, which are generally closely related to the anterior and posterior surfaces of the major calyceal infundibula and the necks of minor calyces. An oblique tract, on the other hand, may damage a significant vessel.[6] Infundibular entry risks injury to interlobar (infundibular) arteries. Access into an anterior calyx or any calyx that does not afford direct access to the stone invites overly aggressive torquing of the sheath and rigid endoscope, which also can lead to hemorrhage. If direct access cannot be obtained, then flexible instrumentation should be considered.[5]

- Additionally, misuse of any tool like lithotrites, resectoscopes, wires, sheaths, graspers, baskets can also cause hemorrhage.

- The access sheath provides intraoperative tamponade of parenchymal bleeding. Postoperatively, hemostasis is achieved by collapse of the parenchyma onto itself. Unless the postoperative nephrostomy tube is as large as or larger than the sheath used during the procedure, it likely does not contribute to hemostasis. There is no difference in measures of postoperative bleeding between no drainage tubes, small (8 to 18 Fr) and large (20 to 28 Fr) drainage tubes.[10–12]

Factors Affecting Blood Loss

Factors associated with hemorrhage during percutaneous renal surgery include patient characteristics, multiple access sites, supra-costal access, increasing tract size, prolonged operative time, and renal pelvic perforation.[5–9]

The reason for the increased incidence of vascular injury with upper calyceal puncture may be related to the oblique and longer length of the tract.[9] In many cases the upper calyx was superior to the site of skin puncture even if a supracostal approach was used. Therefore, an oblique and longer tract was needed. Moreover, changing the direction of the tract to reach the renal pelvis may result in injury to the adjacent parenchyma with its vascular supply. Therefore, it is advisable to enter the upper calyx through a straight and

Table 7.3: Transfusion rate according to Amplatz sheath size[13]

Sheath size	No. of patients	Blood transfusion (%)
Small (18 F and below)	271	3 (1.1%)
Medium (24 F and 26 F)	1039	50 (4.8%)
Large (27 F, 28 F, and 30 F)	3533	208 (5.9%)
Largest (32 F, 33 F, and 34 F)	371	45 (12.1%)

In a large multi-institutional study including 5537 patients, the significant factors associated with hemorrhage during percutaneous renal surgery were larger sheath size, prolonged operative time, case load (center volume: low/mid/high), greater stone burden and multiple tracts.[13]

direct tract in line with the upper infundibulum and pelvis.

Technical complications may lead to excessive bleeding. These include pelvicalyceal tears and loss of the access tract. Infundibular tears may occur during tract dilatation or stone manipulation and may be associated with laceration of significant vessels that lie close to the infundibulum. Subsequent instrument manipulation in that area is likely to enlarge the tear and further traumatize the injured vessel, leading to hemorrhage. Staging the procedure in such cases, especially when dealing with complex calculi or when a significant stone burden is yetto be removed, allows the injury to heal and reduces the bloodloss at a subsequent stage.[6] Loss of percutaneous access can lead to loss of tract tamponade and uncontrolled bleeding from the renal parenchyma. Initial guide and safety wires should be placed and secured carefully.

Clinical Presentation

In a large series conducted by Kessaris,[14] of 0.8% of 2200 patients requiring treatment for hemorrhage after percutaneous renal surgery, 24% of the hemorrhages occurred within 24 hours of surgery, 41% between 2 and 7 days after surgery, and 35% more than 7 days later.

A. Intraoperative and Perioperative Bleeding

- Venous bleeding is generally self-limiting and less likely to be associated with hemodynamic instability. Maneuvers like proper positioning of Amplatz sheath to tamponade the bleeding vessel and increasing the pressure of the irrigating fluid help overcome the bleeding and continue the procedure.

- A significant arterial bleeding is more likely to be associated with fall in blood pressure, hemodynamic instability and poor vision necessitating staging of the procedure.

- A significant vessel bleeding would manifest in many ways like bleeding through and around the nephrostomy tube, clots in the bladder with clot retention, hemodynamic instability (fall in blood pressure, tachycardia, fall in urine output), perinephric hematoma and hypovolemic shock.

- Intraoperative hemorrhage from an injured vein or artery within the collecting system mandates cessation of the procedure if vision deteriorates and/or hemodynamic instability is present. In most cases, especially if the injury appears to be venous, then placing a nephrostomy tube and letting the collecting system clot off is effective.

B. Postoperative Hemorrhage

- Postoperative hemorrhage can occur with the nephrostomy tube in place, at time of tube removal, or afterdischarge from the hospital. Approximately 1% of major percutaneous procedures are complicated by delayed hemorrhage requiring treatment. In a systematic review of reports including a total of 11,929 patients, a 0.4% rate of delayed hemorrhage requiring treatment was reported.[3] This may be exacerbated by strenuous activity, infection or restarting anticoagulation therapy.

- Delayed hemorrhage is usually a result of arteriovenous fistulas or arterial pseudo-aneurysms, with the latter being more common. The lacerated artery is a high pressure system and willleak into a lower pressure system: A vein (fistula) or the parenchyma or hilar areolar tissue (pseudoaneurysm).

- Arteriovenous fistulas occur when a paired set of artery and vein is injured, and arterial blood enters directly into the vein. The weak vein wall cannot sustain the high arterial pressure and ruptures. Bleeding into the collecting system is most commonly noted, but it can be outside the kidney as well. The latter should be suspected if the hematocrit falls but the urine remains relatively clear. It can be confirmed with CT or ultrasonography.

- An arterial pseudoaneurysm occurs when an artery is injured, clots off, and then intermittently ruptures, often clotting off again at variable intervals. Continuous bleeding suggests an arteriovenous fistula, and intermittent bleeding suggests arterial pseudoaneurysm, but the distinction is not critical because treatment is the same.

- Any report of bright red blood in the urine after percutaneous renal surgery should prompt a hospital admission and consi-deration of angiography, which is diagnostic in more than 90% of cases.[14]

- Richstone et al[15] reviewed their data of 4695 percutaneous renal surgeries. 57 of these underwent angiography. The most common findings were renal arterial pseudo-aneurysm (47%), contrast extravasation from a lacerated renal vessel (22%) and arteriovenous fistula (22%). Renal arterial dissection was seen in two patients and one instance each of a hypervascular area, a vascular "cut-off" sign, and a fistula

between an arterial branch and the percutaneous tract were identified. 17.5% patients had more than one lesion. These included patients with staghorn calculi and multiple tract procedures. Venous injuries can be under diagnosed by angiography and may also explain those situations without demonstrable findings. Fortunately, hemorrhage of venous origin usually responds well to conservative management.

- The standard treatment of renal arterio-venous fistulae and arterial pseudoaneu-rysms is selective angioembolization, which is highly effective.

Management

Flowchart 7.1 gives a broad guideline to approach and management of intraoperative bleeding.

Management of Venous Hemorrhage

- Commonly, intraoperative bleeding during PCNL is venous in origin. Maneuvers like increasing the irrigating fluid pressure and placement of an Amplatz sheath may tamponade the parenchymal bleeding and allows the urologist to continue the procedure.

- If placement of the sheath and removal of clots does not restore vision, then one should place and clamp alarge (20–24 Fr) re-entry nephrostomy tube to facilitate clotting and hemostasis.[6, 16] Staging the procedure in such cases, especially when dealing with complex calculi or when a significant stone burden is yet to be removed, allows the injury to heal and reduces the blood loss at a subsequent stage.[6] The second stage surgery should be planned once the patient is hemodyna-mically stable with clear urine from the nephrostomy tube and per urethral catheter and after a minimum of 48 hours delay.

- Minimal tract dilatation and limiting the procedure time help in limiting the renal trauma.

Flowchart 7.1: Approach and management of intraoperative bleeding

Intraoperative bleeding

Increase irrigating fluid pressure
Adjust the Amplatz or nephroscope sheath
Assess hemodynamic status

Vision improves
Hemodynamically stable

Bleeding persistent and/or
hemodynamically unstable

Continue procedure with
hemodynamic monitoring

Infuse IV fluids and colloids rapidly
Assess remaining stone burden or time
required to complete the procedure

If procedure near completion: Clear
the remaining stones and insert a
nephrostomy tube and clamp it

If significant stone burden remaining:
Insert a nephrostomy tube and clamp it.
Stage the procedure

- Postoperatively assess blood loss by fall in Hb and hematocrit
- Monitor: BP, pulse, color and volume of urine from per urethral catheter
- USG for perinephric collection and clots in PCS/bladder
- Declamp nephrostomy tube 4–6 hours later and assess for color of
  drainage through it. If fresh bleeding, reclamp it and declamp 24 hours later

Clear urine from per urethral
catheter and nephrostomy tube,
hemodynamically stable

Clear urine from per urethral
catheter with persistent hemorrhagic
drainage from nephrostomy tube,
hemodynamically stable

Hemodynamically unstable or
persistent hemorrhagic urine
through per urethral and
nephrostomy tubes with or
without clots in bladder and
falling hemoglobin
and hematocrit

Second stage PCNL after
a minimum gap of 48 hours

Check position of nephrostomy
tube. It may have slipped out
partially with tip abutting
against the renal parenchyma

Angiography

Remove nephrostomy and observe for 48 hours. If clinically stable with
clear urine output and no peri- or infrarenal collection and experienced
surgeon, proceed for second stage PCNL through separate calyx of entry

- If hemorrhage continues, a Councill tip or a Kaye tamponade balloon catheter can be inflated in the renal parenchyma to tamponade the venous bleeding. This 36 Fr occlusive balloon is inserted over a 5 F ureteral stent. It has an internal 14 F lumen that allows drainage of the renal pelvis. The Kaye catheter tamponades the nephrostomy tract but also effectively drains the renal pelvis and maintains ureteral access.[16]
- Postoperative strict monitoring is mandatory with pulse and blood pressure recordings, urine output and colour and drop in Hb/hematocrit. Regular ultrasonography may be done to assess presence of pelvicalyceal or perinephric clots and collections.

Management of Arterial Hemorrhage

Significant arterial injury can present with acute or delayed hemorrhage postoperatively. It may present with gross hematuria with or without clots, dizziness, and/or hypovolemic shock.

A small arterial injury can sometimes be addressed intraoperatively with fulguration under direct vision.

After stabilization with crystalloids and blood products, patients should undergo renal angiography and superselective embolization. The rate of postoperative hemorrhage necessitating angioembolization has been reported at 0.8% to 1.3%.[14, 15] In a series of 4,695 patients who underwent PCNL for various indications, Richstone and colleagues reported that 1.2% of patients postoperatively needed angioembolization.[15]

In a multi-institutional review of 10 sites, renal angioembolization as a therapeutic intervention in the management of renal trauma had a success rate of 90%.[17]

Indications for angiography and possible embolization include

- Gross hematuria with clots
- Decreasing hematocrit that does not respond to conservative management.
- Persistent/recurrent hypotension
- Bleeding through nephrostomy
- Clots in bladder/perinephric growing hematoma
- Failed conservative treatment
- Vascular shock

Risks of angiography and angioembolisation

- During selective angiography and embolization, there is a risk of arterial dissection, arterial perforation, and "nontarget" embolization. Nontarget embolization can occur with migration of the embolization medium, such as alcohol, coils, gel foam, glue, or particles.
- Postinfarction syndrome including flank pain, nausea and vomiting is seen in majority of the patients and is self-limiting.

- Contrast-induced nephropathy (CIN) and embolisation-induced loss of renal parenchyma are the important consequences of renal angiography. These are directly related to the amount of contrast injected. Diabetics and patients with renal insufficiency are at higher risk. Protective maneuvers include intravenous hydration and N-acetyl cysteine (NAC) are given 1.2 gm twice a day-to-day prior and on the day of procedure.[16]

Nephrectomy may be required if selective angioembolization fails, and partial or total renal loss may occur if angioembolization is not selective enough.

Management of Perinephric Hematoma

After PCNL, a perinephric hematoma is a common finding. Extracorporeal shock wave lithotripsy before PCNL increases the risk for development of a perinephric hematoma. This is usually clinically insignificant. Decreasing hematocrit despite a clear urine output should raise suspicion of a significant perinephric hematoma. The diagnosis is confirmed with an ultrasound or CT scan. If conservative measures fail, then renal angiography and superselective embolization should be performed in an attempt to identify and embolize the bleeding arterial branches. Once the hematoma liquefies, a percutaneous drain could be placed.

Role of Tranexamic Acid

- Tranexamic acid is a synthetic derivative of the amino acid lysine with strong affinity for 5 lysine binding sites of plasminogen. It acts as an antifibrinolytic which competitively inhibits the activation of plasminogen to plasmin, a molecule responsible for the degradation of fibrin. Fibrin is the basic framework for the formation of blood clot during hemostasis.
- Kumar and colleagues demonstrated reduced blood loss, reduced transfusion rate and reduced operative time in patients

receiving tranexamic acid (1 gm tranexamic acid at induction followed by 3 oral doses of 500 mg during 24 hours) as compared to control patients who did not receive the drug.[18]

- The evidence that tranexamic acid reduces the need for blood transfusion is strong but the safety of routine use of tranexamic acid in surgical patients remains uncertain. A modest increase in the risk of thromboembolic effects could outweigh the benefits of reduced blood loss.[19] Although some increased risk might be expected on theoretical grounds, recent evidence from the clinical randomisation of an antifibrinolytic in significant hemorrhage 2 (CRASH-2) trial of tranexamic acid in bleeding trauma patients showed a statistically significant reduction in mortality with no increase in thromboembolic effects. Indeed, there was a statistically significant reduction in the risk of myocardial infarction in trauma patients who received tranexamic acid.[20, 21]

VISCERAL INJURY

Any abdominal organ close to the kidney can be injured during percutaneous renal surgery including the colon, duodenum, jejunum, spleen, liver, and biliary system.

COLON INJURY

Colonic perforation occurs during percutaneous renal surgery in the prone position at a rate of less than 1%.[5] This low incidence is likely the result of the colon rarely being retrorenal (reported in approximately 0.6% of the general population).[22, 23] As one would expect based on the anatomy, with the apposition of the colon to the kidney being greatest on the left side and at the lower pole, the left colon is injured twice as often as the right colon, and the majority of colon injuries involve access to the lower pole.[24, 25] A puncture site laterally may increase the risk of colon injury. The position of the colon is usually anterior or anterolateral to the lateral renal border.

Therefore, risk of colon injury usually exists only with a very lateral (lateral to the posterior axillary line) puncture.

Risk factors: Displacement of the colon posterior to the kidney increases the risk of colon perforation, and is seen in elderly patients with chronic constipation or patients with other causes of colonic distension, patients with previous major abdominal surgery (jejunoileal bypass, partial jejunoileal bypass), neurologic impairment, and institutional bowel resulting in an enlarged colon. Others at greater risk include thin female patients with a little retroperitoneal fat, and patients with mobile kidneys, anterior calyceal puncture, previous extensive renal surgery, horseshoe kidney and other forms of renal fusion or ectopia and kyphoscoliosis.[23, 24]

Injury might be less likely with the patient in the supine position; one study reported a retrorenal colon on CT in 1.9% of patients in the supine position versus 10% in prone patients.[26] The clinical incidence of colon injury, however, is much lower than this.

Diagnosis

Intraoperative detection of colonic injury confers easier management. Intraoperative detection is difficult. Movement of bowel gas along with the puncture needle and dilators on fluoroscopy should raise suspicion of a trans-colonic tract. Gas escaping out of the puncture site on removal of Amplatz sheath at the end of procedure also hints towards a bowel injury.

If not determined intraoperatively, colon injury should be considered postoperatively if a patient develops unexplained fever, prolonged ileus, unexplained leukocytosis, rectal bleeding, evidence of peritoneal inflammation, or fecaluria or pneumaturia. Clinically apparent nephrocolonic fistula may be the presenting sign, or the injury may not be noted until the time of postoperative nephrostogram. CT imaging is recommended to assess for unsuspected abdominal or retroperitoneal complications that contribute to sepsis, such as colonic perforation.

Treatment

Most colon injuries are extraperitoneal and can be managed conservatively. The main principle of care is prompt and separate drainage of the colon and urinary collecting system. The surgeon should withdraw the offending nephrostomy tube into the colon to serve as a colostomy tube, consider exchanging it for a larger tube to enhance colonic drainage, and obtain separate access to the upper urinary tract with a retrograde-placed ureteral double-J stent. Administer broad-spectrum antibiotics. Give nothing by mouth for a few days, and then start clear liquids. If there is no increase of colostomy output, then administer high-calorie protein supplementation and eventually a regular diet. This allows the renal collecting system and the medial colonic wall to heal within 5–7 days. Confirm lack of communication between the colon and collecting system with contrast injection of the tubes before removing or withdrawing them. The colonic tube should be initially withdrawn slightly and maintained as a drain outside the colon. 3 days later when the lateral colonic wall has healed, the tube can be removed completely.[23]

If the injury is intraperitoneal, or if the patient develops peritonitis or sepsis, then open surgical repair with colostomy may be required.

Small intestine injury: The second and third portions of the duodenum may be injured during percutaneous renal surgery because they are adjacent to the right kidney, but this represents a very rare complication of PCNL and is rarer than colonic perforation. This can occur when the renal pelvis is perforated during dilation, or during placement of the working sheath or stone removal. This complication can be avoided with careful fluoroscopic monitoring during access, tract dilation, working sheath placement, and proper endoscopic manipulations. Injury should be suspected if intestinal mucosa or contents are visualized or if communication with the small bowel is demonstrated on a nephrostogram or on the formation of a nephroduodenal fistula, which is also seen when postoperative nephrostography is obtained. In the face of a large perforation or patient instability, open surgical repair is necessary. For patients with small injuries of the small bowel and no signs of peritonitis or sepsis; however, nonoperative management may be attempted. For this group, antibiotics are administered and bowel rest is achieved with nasogastric suction and parenteral hyperalimentation. The nephrostomy tube should be positioned correctly to assure adequate drainage. Nephrostography and upper gastrointestinal radiography are performed 10–15 days after injury to assess for closure of the fistula.[23, 27, 28]

Liver and Spleen

Studies based on CT and MRI have suggested that splenic and hepatic injuries should be unlikely when the kidney is accessed below the 12th rib, although access above the 11th or 12th rib might traverse these organs in rare cases.[29, 30] Hopper and Yakes performed CT at both maximal inspiration and expiration with sagittal reconstructions in 43 randomly selected patients.[29] They found that the liver and spleen were not in contact with the supra-12th tract, but if the supracostal puncture was performed above the 11th rib during full expiration, the liver was punctured in 14% of cases. The potential risk for splenic and hepatic injury is significant during access above the 11th rib. A site of skin puncture as medial as possible, is mandatory to avoid direct damage to the spleen and the liver.[30]

If splenomegaly or hepatomegaly is present, these relationships change and access guided by CT is recommended. Splenic or hepatic injuries to orthotopic and normal-sized organs occur almost exclusively with supracostal upper pole renal access. Splenic injury might require laparotomy and potentially splenectomy owing to hemorrhage, but conservative management has been successful as well. Liver injury is less likely to be associated with significant hemorrhage. Liver injuries during percutaneous renal surgery can be managed conservatively.[31] There have been a few reported cases of biliary peritonitis resulting from injury of the gallbladder or biliary tree, which require exploratory laparotomy/laparoscopy and cholecystectomy owing to the high mortality rate of bile peritonitis.

THORACIC COMPLICATIONS

Thoracic complications include pneumothorax, hydrothorax, hemothorax, and nephropleural fistula, with the possibility of more than one of these conditions coexisting. The incidence of these complications ranges from 0 to 18%, varying in part due to the type of renal access obtained.[32–37]

Pathophysiology

- Pneumothorax can occur via the introduction of air into the pleural space while obtaining access or during the procedure, and to a lesser degree during nephrostomy tube removal. Alternatively, an injury to the lung can also result in a tension pneumothorax.

- Hydrothorax can occur during the procedure when irrigation fluid or urine enters the pleural space along the nephrostomy tract or from diaphragmatic irritation with a reactive effusion. Occasionally, hydrothorax can have a delayed occurrence from urine that leaks through the PCNL tract in the pleural space.

- Hemothorax is usually the result of an injury to the intercostal artery, diaphragm, renal parenchyma, or renal vasculature, with subsequent bleeding into the pleural space. Similar to the pathophysiology of hydrothorax, bleeding from the kidney can also track along the nephrostomy tube tract into the pleural space.

- Nephropleural fistula results from the persistent drainage of urine from the renal collecting system into the pleural space and is similar to hydrothorax. While hydrothorax usually presents early in the postoperative course due to fluid collection during or shortly after the procedure, a nephropleural fistula often occurs later after nephrostomy tube removal. Development of a nephropleural fistula may be associated with distal collecting system obstruction.

- Empyema is usually neglected pleural effusion, or if a supracostal access was used in the presence of urinary infection or pyonephrosis.

Anatomic Details

The pleura, a thin and serous membrane that covers the lung and the chest wall, is divided in two anatomic layers—the visceral and the parietal. The visceral layer envelops the lung parenchyma, while the parietal layer covers the ribs, diaphragm, and mediastinum. The virtual cavity between these two layers is the pleural space. Under normal circumstances, the pleural surfaces are tightly coapted, and the cavity contains only a small amount of fluid. Stening and Bourne have discussed in depth the anatomic considerations in the supracostal approach for renal surgery.[34] The lower limit of the parietal pleura crosses the 12th rib obliquely at its midpoint such that the lateral half of the rib is uncovered by the pleura. In the midscapular line, the visceral pleura is in relation to the 10th rib, while the parietal pleura is at the level of the 12th rib. The parietal and visceral pleurae ascend cranially and laterally on the ribs, and further rise in deep expiration (Fig. 7.1). Thus, a puncture made lateral to the midscapular line, below the 10th rib, in deep expiration would almost always prevent damage to the visceral pleura. Tracts below the 11th rib made lateral to the midscapular line would miss not only the visceral

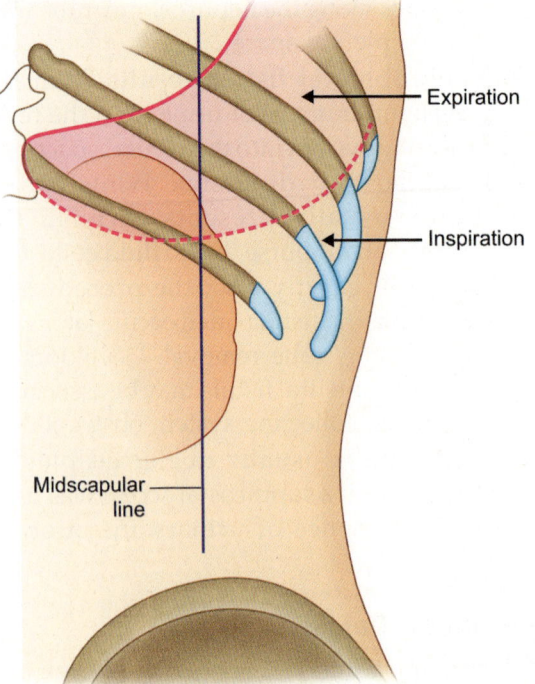

Expiration

Inspiration

Midscapular
line

Fig. 7.1: Diagrammatic representation of parietal pleura during phases of respiration

pleura but also may miss the parietal pleura. Tracts made through the parietal pleura may not be of clinical significance, especially when the Amplatz sheath is used, because this would avoid the leakage of the irrigation fluid in the pleural space by maintaining a low-pressure irrigation.

Diagnosis

The pleural violation can be diagnosed immediately after PCNL or may be seen in the immediate postoperative period. Late presentation is very unusual.

- Fluoroscopic examination of the chest should be a protocol in every patient when supracostal access is used. A clear costophrenic angle (CPA) rules out any pleural violation. When CPA is obscured, pleural injury is suspected, and further evaluation is considered.[33] Patients who have a clear CPA are followed by clinical examination and chest auscultation in the postoperative period.

- Chest radiography (both postero-anterior and lateral views) should be performed to confirm any suspicious finding on clinical examination. In patients who have undergone asupracostal puncture, irrespective of auscultation findings, radiographic documentation of a normal pleural space should be performed after nephrostomy tube removal.

- Ultrasonography of the lower chest may discover more patients with a small fluid collection. As little as 50 ml of fluid can be visualized on ultrasonography, while radiography would only detect fluid more than 250 ml. Lateral decubitus chest radiography will allow smaller amounts of fluid to be detected.

- In the postoperative period, the diagnosis of a thoracic complication is often based on the patient's symptoms. Complaints may include shortness of breath or chest pain, with objective findings including increasing oxygen requirement and decreased breath sounds over the affected lung field.

- Kekre et al presented their series of 102 supracostal PCNL procedures wherein 10 patients were diagnosed with thoracic complications. Four patients were diagnosed intraoperatively before extubation, three were diagnosed in the recovery room based on oxygen saturations and three developed shortness of breath and tachypnea several hours later after transfer to the surgical ward.[36]

- Late occurrence of a symptomatic chest collection is very rare, especially if the radiograph after nephrostomy tube removal was documented as normal. Late pleural effusion is possible in patients who have a double-J stent in place. Bladder spasms with high-pressure stent-related reflux might lead to a leak of bladder urine into the pleural space through the healing PCNL tract. In patients, who do not have a DJ stent, a leak in the plcural space could be caused by ureteral obstruction from a small residual fragment or post-procedure edema.

- Nephropleural fistula may present later after nephrostomy tube removal with persistent drainage from the chest tube placed for hydrothorax. A retrograde pyelogram may be necessary to document a fistulous connection between the collecting system and pleural space after supracostal PCNL. Causes include obstructed or improperly positioned DJ stent or distal ureteral obstruction, which can be assessed with a retrograde ureteropyelogram.

Prevention

1. At the beginning of the procedure, fluoroscopic evaluation can assist in identifying the inferior pleural margin. Biplanar fluoroscopy may provide superior visualization of the anatomic relationship between the kidney and pleural space, and decrease the risk of complications.[32]
2. Supracostal access should be performed lateral to the midscapular line to minimize injury to the pleura.[32–34]
3. The needle should be advanced along the upper margin of the rib during the expiratory phase. Needle passage along the inferior margin of the rib risks injury to the intercostal neurovascular bundle, which can result in significant bleeding.
4. The supracostal skin puncture should be done over the lateral portion of the rib, and the puncture should be made during steady, quiet breathing or breath holding in expiration. However, the calyceal entry can be made during full inspiration when the kidney descends caudally.[38]
5. Pedro et al describe a technique of renal displacement to allow the renal access to be obtained more caudally than would otherwise be possible.[39] If the targeted calyx is above the 11th rib, the authors place an extra access site into a mid-posterior calyx to help displace the kidney caudally. This access site can also be used for postoperative drainage.

6. Once access has been obtained and the tract dilated, an Amplatz access sheath should be placed to minimize extravasation of irrigant into the retroperitoneum and pleural space. In the event that the parietal pleura is traversed by the needle, the use of an access sheath can often prevent this from evolving into a thoracic complication.
7. The amount of irrigant used during the procedure should be monitored, although a precise measurement is difficult. If the inflow of irrigant is significantly more than the measured outflow, the possibility of extravasation into the pleural space should be considered, and the chest fluoroscopically evaluated.
8. If a nephrostomy tube is left at the end of the procedure, the appropriate position within the collecting system is of importance. An antegrade nephrostogram can help to ensure that the catheter is well-positioned. Shaban et al described a case of a nephropleural fistula 2 days after PCNL in a patient with dyspnea, chest pain, and fever.[35] An antegrade nephrostogram demonstrated one side-hole of the nephrostomy tube to be outside of the kidney, with extravasation of urine into the pleural space. The patient was managed with a thoracostomy tube and an internal ureteral stent.

Management

- All patients with supracostal access should be regarded as high risk for thoracic complications.
- At the conclusion of each percutaneous renal surgery procedure, the lung field and costophrenic sulcus should be closely evaluated with fluoroscopy. A relatively small pleural effusion or pneumothorax noted on intraoperative fluoroscopy, in the absence of any changes in ventilatory parameters, may be managed conservatively or with simple needle aspiration. When a large pleural effusion or pneumothorax is noted intraoperatively, a thoracostomy

tube should be placed with the patient under anesthesia.

- In the postoperative period, the management of hydrothorax depends on the size of the effusion and the degree to which the patient is affected. Minimal blunting of the costophrenic angle can usually be managed conservatively.[32, 33] Large or symptomatic effusions should be treated with drainage of the pleural space. Needle aspiration can relieve a smaller effusion, but tube thoracostomy should be used for larger effusions. The thoracostomy output and CXR are monitored, and with resolution of drainage and the effusion, the tube can be removed. The average duration of chest drainage is 3–4 days.[32] If a second-look PCNL is planned, the thoracostomy tube should be left in place until after this procedure is completed.

- In patients with a late presentation of pleural effusion presence of properly positioned DJ stent needs to be confirmed. In the presence of a stent, the collection could be from stent-related reflux; hence, this is managed by keeping the bladder empty with an indwelling Foley catheter and preventing bladder spasms with anticholinergic drugs. In the absence of a stent, the collection could be from a small calculus fragment or blood clot that is blocking the ureter. This is managed by placing a DJ stent to be obstruct the kidney.[3] The Foley catheter is kept inplace until drainage stops from the chest tube.

- Complications can develop in the setting of an undrained or poorly drained hemothorax. These include empyema and fibrothorax. Early evacuation of a hemothorax is critical to decrease the risk of these complications. The goal of early drainage is to prevent formation of loculations, which occur approximately 7 days after the initial injury.

- Tubeless PCNL: Tubeless percutaneous nephrolithotomy is likely safe in appropriately selected patients, and with close

attention paid to fluoroscopic evaluation of the lung field and costophrenic angle at the completion of the procedure. Shah et al described 454 tubeless PCNL procedures using 535 renal tracts, of which 358 were supracostal.[40] The authors found that tubeless PCNL was not associated with more chest complications compared to standard PCNL in which a nephrostomy tube is left at the end of the procedure.

POSTOPERATIVE FEVER AND SEPSIS

After percutaneous nephrolithotomy, 15 to 30% of patients develop fever, whereas sepsis occurs in 0.5 to 2.5% of patients.[5] Most cases of fever following PCNL are minor and easily managed without intervention. However, the concerns regarding post-PCNL fever are bacteremia and urinary extravasation, which may develop into septicemia and septic shock that increase morbidity and mortality.

Pathogenesis

Fever following PCNL may be secondary to urinary tract infection (UTI). Bacterial infection from stone or renal pelvic urine may enter the bloodstream during stone manipulation through pyelovenous, pyelolymphatic and pyelotubular back flows and forniceal rupture.[41]

However, fever may also originate from the release of the inflammatory mediators during surgical manipulation—systemic inflammatory response syndrome (SIRS).

A positive urine culture is associated with a two-fold risk of fever in the postoperative period.[42] The risk of postoperative fever among the patients with a positive urine culture depends on the specific micro-organisms found in their urine. Specifically, postoperative fever was reported in 9.7–14.5% of the patients whose urine cultures consisted of Gram-positive micro-organisms (*Staphylococcus* spp. and *Enterococcus* spp.) but in 19.4–23.8% of the patients with Gram-negative micro-organisms (e.g. *E. coli*, *Enterobacter* spp. and others).[42]

A negative urine culture does not guarantee against sepsis because the voided urine culture may not reflect the intrarenal urine. The percentage of post-PCNL fever in patients with negative preoperative urine culture and positive preoperative urine culture was 8.8% and 18.2%, respectively. Positive stone and pelvic urine culture are better predictors of the potential post-PCNL sepsis than bladder urine culture. Mariappan et al in a prospective study showed that the positive predictive value and negative predictive value of preoperative urine cultures were 5% and 56%, respectively. Patients with positive stone and pelvic urine cultures had four times greater risk of urosepsis.[43]

Risk Factors

Factors affecting the risk of postoperative sepsis could be divided into preoperative, intraoperative, and postoperative factors.[41–44]

- Preoperative factors include positive preoperative urine culture, positive intraoperative urine culture, stone size, infected stone, neurogenic bladder dysfunction, diabetes mellitus and abnormality of renal anatomy.
- Intraoperative factors include renal pelvic pressure, operative time, and multiple tracts.
- Postoperative factors include nephrostomy tube placement, urethral catheter placement, and antibiotic administration.

Pus or Turbid Fluid Aspirated on Puncture

- If pus is aspirated upon initial percutaneous entry to the upper urinary tract, the safest measure is to abort the procedure and leave a nephrostomy tube for drainage.
- Incidental aspiration of purulent fluids at the time of renal access is occasionally possible even in situations where there is no fever, bacteremia, or recent UTI. The general practice in such situations is nephrostomy tube placement until sterile urine is obtained, followed by delayed PCNL.

- The purulent fluid found during renal access is however not always infected. Positive fluid cultures are found in fewer than half of these patients. The previous antibiotic usage, a sterile inflammatory tissue in response to calculus and macroscopic crystalline or amorphous calculi may take a role in this condition.
- Hosseini et al[45] reported the efficacy and safety of PCNLs in 45 patients with staghorn renal stones and incidental purulent fluids in the pelvicalyceal system. A total of 29 patients received immediate PCNL, whereas the remaining 16 patients received delayed PCNL (3–5 days later) after nephrostomy tube placement and treatment with antibiotics. In patients, who received immediate and delayed PCNL, 10.3% and 12.5% patients, respectively, experienced low-grade fever for 12–24 hours. The percentages of positive fluid culture and positive stone cultures are not different in both groups. E. coli was the most common organism in both groups followed by Pseudomonas aeruginosa and Klebsiella pneumoniae. The authors concluded that PCNL can be safely performed in this condition with full antibiotic administration.
- Etemadian et al[46] suggested that even if thick pus is aspirated during the initial puncture of PCNL, PCNL can be safely continued using a low-pressure Amplatz sheath and empirical antibiotics. The risk factors of sepsis in these cases were a recent history of UTI, borderline elevation of total leukocyte count, thick foul pus on initial access, multiple tracts, and operative time more than 90 minutes. Patients with these factors should have initial nephrostomy tube drainage, and multiple tracts might be needed to drain all blocked calyces.[45–47]

Prophylactic Antibiotic Administration and Prevention of Infective Complications

- Prophylactic antibiotics are recommended in PCNL procedure because PCNL is a clean-contaminated (uncomplicated stone without obstruction, without stent and without history of UTI) or contaminated (complex stone with obstruction, nephrostomy tube or DJ stent placement) surgical procedure. Despite the negative preoperative urine cultures, perioperative antibiotic is routinely administered and routine bacteriologic evaluation should be performed when postoperative fever occurs. The role of prophylactic antibiotics is to only decrease the risk of postoperative infection complications, and they do not completely eliminate the risk of infection. The European Urologic Association (EAU) guideline recommends prophylactic antibiotic for percutaneous stone surgery due to the high risk of infection following this procedure (Level 1b, Grade A). Patients with infected stones, a recent history of UTI, and a positive urine culture should receive prophylactic antibiotics prior to undergoing PCNL, which should be continued for at least 4 days postoperatively. The guideline also recommends an appropriate prophylactic antibiotic for sterile urine preoperatively as a means of decreasing the incidence of postoperative sepsis.[48] The duration of antibiotic depends on whether the stone is uncomplicated or complex. The optimal drugs are broad-spectrum antibiotics and depend on sensitivity of antibiogram in the hospital.

- Stone culture is the best predictor of urosepsis. A significant difference in the number and type of different pathogens isolated between stone culture and urine culture is demonstrated, which is very important in clinical practice for selection of suitable postoperative antibiotics.[43] The preoperative urine culture is less clinically important, which may be sterile due to the effect of preoperative antibiotics and obstruction of urinary tract.
- Good surgical technique with low intrarenal pressure is also necessary to prevent this

common complication. Monga et al demonstrated that high pressure irrigation statistically (p. 0.0002) increases the risk of SIRS (46% vs 11%).[49] Similarly, Zhong et al reported that the cumulative time (>50 sec) spent with renal pelvic pressure greater than 30 mm Hg contributed to the risk of postoperative fever after PCNL.[50] Dogan et al reported that the most important factors affecting postoperative fever were the duration of surgery and the amount of irrigation fluid used.[51] A higher risk of fever was encountered when these factors exceeded the critical values of 102 minutes operating time or 23 L irrigation fluid.

METABOLIC AND PHYSIOLOGICAL COMPLICATIONS

- Normal saline should be the irrigant for percutaneous renal surgery, with the exception of glycine or similar non-electrolytic isotonic fluids when monopolar electrocautery is used.[5]
- Irrigation with water during percutaneous renal surgery risks intravascular hemolysis, which can be fatal. Intravascular or extravascular extravasation of nonelectrolytic isotonic fluid from continued irrigation in the setting of a large venous injury or collecting system perforation, respectively, can result in hyponatremia and other electrolyte abnormalities, renal or hepatic dysfunction and mental status changes.
- When normal saline is used in uncomplicated cases, the amount of fluid absorption is generally clinically in significant.[52] A large amount of saline extravasation can lead to clinically significant respiratory distress or cardiac failure resulting from volume overload.
- Reducing the height of the irrigating fluid bag and use of an Amplatz open drainage (low pressure) sheath helps keep the intrapelvic pressure low and prevents fluid absorption.

- Major perforations of the pelvicalyceal wall or infundibular tears allow direct access of fluid to the perinephric space and subsequent absorption. In the presence of extravasation or excessive bleeding, the procedure should be terminated and completed later. This reduces the amount of bleeding, allows the tract to mature, and reduces fluid absorption.
- High irrigation pressures increase the risk of systemic inflammatory response syndrome after PCNL. As such, consideration should be given to minimizing irrigation pressures or using intermittent high pressure, particularly in patients a thigh risk for infectious complications.[49, 52]
- Volume of irrigation fluid >20 liters at room temperature was associated with intraoperative hypothermia and cardiovascular changes (blood pressure changes of more than 20% from the baseline).[53]
- Venous gas embolism is a rare but potentially fatal complication of percutaneous renal surgery. The gas (in this case, air) enters the venous system and passes through the right heart into the pulmonary circulation, blocking the output of the right heart, which results in hypoxemia, hypercapnia and depressed cardiac output. Retrograde air pyelography has been reported as a risk factor.[54, 55]

NEUROMUSCULOSKELETAL COMPLICATIONS

Prone positioning for percutaneous renal surgery has the potential for a number of neuromusculoskeletal injuries.[5, 56] Excessive pressure on neural and vascular structures, whether directly from the operative table or indirectly through the positioning of limbs, may lead to short- or long-term disability.

Most reported injuries associated with prone positioning are related to the head and neck region including ocular injury resulting in visual loss, facial nerve injury or necrosis over facial bones or the tip of the nose, and cerebrovascular accident resulting from carotid or vertebrobasilar artery dissection. Postoperative visual loss (POVL) may occur due to ischemic injury to the optic nerve secondary to venous congestion. Prone position may further increase the intraocular pressure in patients with glaucoma. Other causes of POVL include central retinal artery occlusion, cortical blindness, direct orbital injury and retinal detachment. Blood loss greater than 1,000 ml and duration of anesthesia greater than six hours were identified as strong risk factors. Use of reverse Trendelenburg position and neutral neck position help reducing venous congestion. Routine eye checks every 30 minutes should be done to ensure no direct pressure on the eyes. Hypotension and hypovolemia should also be avoided.

Turning a patient from the supine to the prone position should be performed carefully, avoiding excessive neck movement and allowing normal blood flow in the carotid and vertebral arteries. Careful padding of the head, in a neutral and non-extended position, is important.

There are many reported complications involving the ETT of patients positioned prone, including kinking, obstruction from secretions, migration towards the carina or main stem bronchus, and dislodgement from the patient's trachea. Kinking can occur during hyperflexion of the neck. A reinforced endotracheal tube (ETT) should be considered over a standard ETT.

Malpositioning of the extremities can lead to peripheral nerve injury.[57] The shoulder and elbow should not be abducted more than 90°, so as to prevent brachial plexopathy, and generous padding at the elbow and forearm reduces the risk of nerve compression. Knees need to be padded. Ankles should be elevated to reduce pressure on the dorsum of the foot. Table 7.4 enumerates the body partwise checklist to be taken care of with the possible complications.

Table 7.4: Prone position checklist with possible complications

	Location	Checklist	Possible complications
1.	Eyes	Keep eyes properly taped with no pressure on eyes, nose	Corneal edema, POVL
2.	Tongue	Should be in the mouth and not protruding between the teeth	Macroglossia due to reduced lymphatic and venous drainage
3.	Neck	Maintain 1–2 finger breadths between chest and chin avoiding excessive flexion or extension	Extrinsic airway compression, carotid or vertebral artery dissection, cervical cord injury
4.	Arms	Pad all bony prominences Shoulders and elbows to be abducted <90°	Brachial plexus, ulnar, radial nerve injuries
5.	Chest	Well padded. Breasts should be positioned medial to bolsters	Reduced chest wall compliance with high airway pressures leading to barotrauma, pneumothorax Skin, breast necrosis
6.	Abdomen/ pelvis	Should not be compressed. Bolsters are helpful Avoid pressures on male genitalia Urinary catheter should not be kinked	Compression of IVC causing decreased venous return. High intra-abdominal pressures may lead to increased venous pressure with increased bleeding
7.	Legs	Pad all bony prominences Avoid stretching of nerves Elevate knees to decrease tension on back Elevate ankles so toes are hanging freely	Femoral/sciatic/lateral cutaneous/peroneal nerve injuries Skin ischemia

References

1. Lang, E.K. Percutaneous nephrostolithotomy and lithotripsy:a multi-institutional survey of complications.Radiology 1987;162:25–30.

2. Duvdevani, M., Razvi, H., Sofer, M, et al. Third prize: contemporary percutaneous nephrolithotripsy: 1585 proceduresin 1338 consecutive patients. J Endourol 2007;21:824–29.

3. Seitz C, Desai M, Häcker A, et al. Incidence, prevention, and management of complications following percutaneous nephrolitholapaxy. Eur Urol 2012;61:146–58.

4. Labate G, Modi P, Timoney A, et al. The percutaneous nephrolithotomy global study: classificationof complications. J Endourol 2011;25:1275–80.

5. J Stuart Wolf. Percutaneous Approaches to the Upper UrinaryTract Collecting System. Campbell-Walsh Urology, 11th edition.

6. Kukreja R, Desai M, Patel S, et al. Factors affecting blood loss during percutaneous nephrolithotomy: prospective study. J Endourol 2004;18:715–22.

7. Stoller ML, Wolf JS, St Lezin MA. Estimated blood loss and transfusion rates associated with percutaneous nephrolithotomy. J Urol 1994;152: 1977.

8. Keoghane SR, Cetti RJ, Rogers AE, et al. Blood transfusion, embolisation and nephrectomy afterpercutaneous nephrolithotomy (PCNL). BJU Int 2012;111:628–32.

9. Ahmed R. El-Nahas, Ahmed A. Shokeir, et al. Post-percutaneous Nephrolithotomy Extensive Hemorrhage: A Study of Risk Factors. J Urol 2007; 177: 576.

10. Lu Y, Ping JG, Zhao XJ, et al. Randomized prospective trial of tubeless versus conventional minimally invasive percutaneous nephrolithotomy. World J Urol 2013;31:1303–07.

11. Maheshwari PN, Andankar MG, Bansal M. Nephrostomy tube after percutaneous nephro-lithotomy: large bore or pigtail catheter? J Endourol 2000;14:735–737.

12. Desai MR, Kukreja R, Desai MM, et al. A prospective randomized comparison of type of nephrostomy drainage following percutaneous

nephrostolithotomy: large bore versus small bore versus tubeless. J Urol 2004;172:565–67.

13. Yamaguchi A, Skolarikos A, Buchholz NP, et al.Operating times and bleeding complications inpercutaneous nephrolithotomy: a comparison of tract dilation methods in 5,537 patients in the Clinical Research Office of the Endourological Society Percutaneous Nephrolithotomy Global Study. J Endourol. 2011;25:933–39.

14. Kessaris DN, Bellman GC, Pardalidis NP, et al. Management of hemorrhage after percutaneous renal surgery. J Urol 1995;153:604–08.

15. Richstone L, Reggio E, Ost MC, et al. Hemorrhage following percutaneous renal surgery: characterization of angiographic findings. J Endourol 2008;22:1129–35.

16. Ardeshir R, Smith AD, Siegel DN, et al. Management of Hemorrhagic Complications associated with Percutaneous Nephrolithotomy. J Endourol 2009;23:1763–67.

17. Breyer BN, McAninch JW, Elliott SP, Master VA. Minimallyinvasive endovascular techniques to treat acute renal hemorrhage. J Urol 2008;179: 2248–53.

18. Santosh Kumar, Singh SK, et al. Tranexamic acid reduces blood loss during percutaneous nephrolithotomy: a prospective randomized controlled study. J Urol 2013 May;189(5):1757–61.

19. Ker K, Edwards P, et al. Effect of tranexamic acid on surgical bleeding: systematic review and cumulative meta-analysis. BMJ 2012;344:e3054.

20. The CRASH-2 Collaborators. Effects of tranexamic acid on death, vascular occlusive events, and blood transfusion in trauma patients with significant haemorrhage (CRASH-2):a randomised, placebo-controlled trial. Lancet 2010;376:23–32.

21. Myles PS, Smith J, Knight J, Cooper DJ, Silbert B, McNeil J, et al. Aspirin and TranexamicAcid for Coronary Artery Surgery (ATACAS) Trial: rationale and design. Am Heart J 2008;155:224–30.

22. Sherman, J.L., Hopper, K.D., Greene, A.J., Johns, T.T. Theretrorenal colon on computed tomography: A normal variant. J Comput Assist Tomogr 1985;9:339–41.

23. Traxer O and Qahtani S. Bowel and other organ injury during percutaneous renal surgery. Smith's Textbook of Endourology, third edition.

24. El-Nahas AR, Shokeir AA, El-Assmy AM, et al. Colonic perforation during percutaneous nephrolithotomy: study of risk factors. Urology 2006;67:937–41.

25. Kachrilas S, Papatsoris A, Bach C, et al. Colon perforation during percutaneous renal surgery: a 10-year experience in a single endourology centre. Urol Res 2012;40:263–68.

26. Hopper KD, Sherman JL, Luethke JM, et al. The retrorenal colon in the supine and prone patient. Radiology 1987;162:443–46.

27. Culkin, D.J., Wheeler, J.S. Jr, Canning, J.R. Nephroduodenal fistula: A complication of percutaneous nephrolithotomy. J Urol 1985;134: 528–30.

28. Duvdevani, M., Razvi, H., Sofer, M. et al. Third prize: Contemporary percutaneous nephrolithotripsy: 1585 procedures in 1338 consecutive patients. J Endourol 2007;21:824–29.

29. Hopper, K.D., Yakes, W.F. The posterior intercostal approach for percutaneous renal procedures: Risk of puncturing the lung, spleen, and liver as determined by CT. AJR Am J Roentgenol 1990;154:115–17.

30. Robert M, Maubon A, Roux JO, et al. Direct percutaneous approach to the upper pole of the kidney: MRI anatomy with assessment of the visceral risk. J Endourol 1999;13:17–20.

31. El-Nahas, A.R., Mansour, A.M., Ellaithy, R., Abol-Enein, H. Case report: conservative treatment of liver injury during percutaneous nephrolithotomy. J Endourol 2008;22:1649–52.

32. Yates J, Munver R. Diagnosis and Management of Thoracic Complications of Percutaneous Renal Surgery. Smith's Textbook of Endourology, third edition.

33. Maheshwari PN, Mane DA, Pathak AB. Management of pleural injury after percutaneous renal surgery. J Endourol 2009;23:1769–72.

34. Stening SG, Bourne S. Supracostal percutaneous nephrolithotomy for upper pole calyceal calculi. J Endourol 1998;12:359–62.

35. Shaban A, Kodera A, El Ghoneimy MN, et al. Safety and efficacy of supracostal access in percutaneous renal surgery.J Endourol 2008;22:29–34.

36. Kekre NS, Gopalakrishnan GG, Gupta GG, Abraham BN, Sharma E. Supracostal approach in percutaneous nephrolithotomy: Experience with 102 cases. J Endourol 2001;15:789–91.

37. Munver R., Delvecchio FC, Newman GE, Preminger G.M. Critical analysis of supracostal access for percutaneous renal surgery. J Urol 2001;166:1242–46.

38. El-Nahas AR, Shokeir AA, El-Kenawy M.R. et al. Safety and efficacy of supracostal percutaneous nephrolithotomy in pediatric patients. J Urol 2008;180:676–80.

39. Pedro RN, Netto NR. Upper-pole access for percutaneous nephrolithotomy. J Endourol 2009;23:1645–47.

40. Shah H, Khandkar A, Sodha H, Kharodawala S, Hedge S, Bansal M. Tubeless percutaneous nephrolithotomy: 3 years of experience with 454 patients. BJU Int 2009;104:840–46.

41. Lojanapiwat B. Infective complication following percutaneous nephrolithotomy. Urological Science 2016;27:8–12.

42. Gutierrez J, Smith A, Geavlete P, et al. Urinary tract infections and postoperative fever in percutaneous nephrolithotomy. World J Urol 2013;31:1135–40.

43. Mariappan P, Smith G, Bariol SV, et al. Stone and pelvic urine culture and sensitivity are better than bladder urine as predictors of urosepsis following percutaneous nephrolithotomy: a prospective clinical study. J Urol 2005;173:1610–14.

44. Healy KA, Ogan K. Pathophysiology and management of infectious staghorn calculi. Urol Clin North Am 2007;34:363e–74.

45. M.M. Hosseini, A. Basiri, S.M. Moghaddam. Percutaneous nephrolithotomy of patients with staghorn stone and incidental purulent fluid suggestive of infection. J Endourol 2007;21: 1429–1432.

46. M. Etemadian, R. Haghighi, A. Madineay, A. Tizeno, S.M. Fereshtehnejad. Delayed versus same-day percutaneous nephrolithotomy in patients with aspirated cloudy urine. Urol J 2008;5:28–33.

47. Aron M, Goel R, Gupta NP, Seth A. Incidental detection of purulent fluid in kidney at percutaneous nephrolithotomy for branched renal calculi. J Endourol 2005;19:136–39.

48. Grabe M, Bartoletti R, Bjerklund-Johansen TE, Çek HM, Pickard RS, Tenke P, et al. Guidelines on urological infections. Arnhem, Netherlands: European Association of Urology; 2014.

49. Omar M, Monga M, et al. Systemic Inflammatory Response Syndrome after Percutaneous Nephrolithotomy: A Randomized Single-Blind Clinical Trial Evaluating the Impact of Irrigation Pressure. J Urol 2016;196:109–14.

50. Zhong W, Zeng G, Wu K, et al. Does a smaller tract in percutaneous nephrolithotomy contribute to high renal pelvic pressure and postoperative fever? J Endourol 2008;22:2147.

51. Dogan HS, Sahin A, Cetinkaya Y, et al. Antibiotic prophylaxis in percutaneous nephrolithotomy: prospective study in 81 patients. J Endourol 2002; 16:649.

52. Kukreja RA, Desai MR, Sabnis RB, et al. Fluid absorption during percutaneous nephrolithotomy: does it matter? J Endourol 2002;16:221–24.

53. Vorrakitpokatorn P, et al. Perioperative Complications and Risk Factors of PCNL. J Med Assoc Thai 2006; 89 (6): 826–33.

54. Song SH, Hong B, Park HK, et al. Paradoxical air embolism during percutaneous nephrolithotomy: a case report. J Korean Med Sci 2007;22:1071–73.

55. Varkarakis J, Su LM, Hsu TH. Air embolism from pneumopyelography. J Urol 2003;169:267.

56. Edgcombe H, Carter K, Yarrow S. Anaesthesia in the prone position. Br J Anaesth 2008;100:165–83.

57. Winfree CJ, Kline DG. Intraoperative positioning nerve injuries. Surg Neurol 2005;63:5–18.

58. Chui J, Craen RA. An update on prone position: Continuing Professional Development. Can J Anesth 2016;63:737–67.

8 | PCNL for Staghorn Calculi

Rajesh Kukreja

PCNL monotherapy is the standard recommendation for staghorn calculi.[1,2] Staghorn calculi due to their large burden, complex configuration and chronicity lead to altered renal function and increased association with infection and hence present a challenging scenario. Complete stone removal should be the goal to reduce chances of future recurrences and infection and preserve renal function.[2]

Preoperative Planning

- **CT scan with 3D reconstruction:** Planning a PCNL for staghorn calculi depends on the stone burden and configuration with relation to the pelvicalyceal system. Anatomically, staghorn calculi have been defined as a branched renal calculus extending into few or all of the calyces.[2] A partial staghorn defines a renal calculus extending into 2 calyces; whereas a complete staghorn defines a calculus extending into all of the calyces and occupying at least 80% of the volume of the pelvicalyceal system. Planning a PCNL does not only depend upon the calculus burden. It needs to take into account the volume and configuration of the stone as well as that of the pelvicalyceal system. The primary tract has to be one that can give access to pelvis and maximum calyces and hence to the maximum stone burden. Secondary tracts would be needed for calyces with calculi unapproachable through the primary tract. CT scan with 3D reconstruction of the stone volume and the pelvicalyceal anatomy helps in planning a PCNL with complex renal disease and achieve higher one stage stone-free rates.[3–6] A morphometry based classification has been proposed by Mishra and colleagues.[7] The classification was made according to the total stone volume (TSV) and unfavorable calyx stone percentile volume (UFCSPV). In order to quantitate the stone volume, CT urography was performed and stone volume was assessed using a CT scan volumetric assessment software. The assessment of favorable and unfavorable calyx was performed on the image plane view of the software. A favorable calyx was defined as a calyx-containing stone that is at an obtuse angle to the entry calyx and has an infundibular width >8 mm. The stones were classified in the following groups. Type 1 staghorn <5000 mm^3 TSV and <5% UFCSPV; Type 2a 5000–20,000 mm^3 TSV and <5% UFCSPV; Type 2b <20,000 mm^3 TSV and >5% UFCSPV; and Type 3 >20,000 mm^3 and any UFCSPV. Multivariate analysis revealed that the tract depends on the UFCSPV while the stages required depend on the TSV in PCNL monotherapy. The combination of TSV and UFCSPV predicted the complexity of staghorn. Similar results were demonstrated by Paul et al.[8] The staghorn morphometry also correlated with stages of PCNL. Increasing stone volume resulted in increasing stages. Unfavorable calyx stone volume and percentile stone volume were higher in multiple tract and multiple stage procedures.

- **Prophylactic antibiotics:** Staghorn calculi are most frequently composed of mixtures of magnesium ammonium phosphate (struvite) and/or calcium carbonate apatite and also referred to as 'infection stones'.[2] Cultures of such stones are generally positive for bacterial growth. In multi-institutional review, stone cultures were positive in 72% of patients with struvite stones.[9] Urea-splitting organisms accounted for only half of the positive stone cultures. *Enterococcus* (9/50, 18%), *Proteus* (9/50, 18%), and *Escherichia coli* (6/50, 12%) were the most commonly identified organisms. Such stones are associated with recurrent infections. PCNL for complex stones is hence considered as a contaminated surgery. The stone size, prolonged operative time, stone culture and multiple tracts are all high risk factors for post-procedural fever and sepsis.[10–13] The European Urologic Association (EAU) guideline recommends prophylactic antibiotic for percutaneous stone surgery due to the high risk of infection following this procedure (level 1b, grade A). Patients with infected stones, a recent history of UTI, and a positive urine culture should receive prophylactic antibiotics prior to undergoing PCNL, which should be continued for at least 4 days post-operatively.[14] The optimal drugs are broad-spectrum antibiotics and depend on sensitivity of antibiogram in the hospital.

Intraoperative Principles

1. **Prepuncturing all the desired calyces:** The primary calyx of entry is selected based on the CT assessment. Intraoperative retrograde pyelography may also help in deciding this.

The primary tract should give access to the majority of the stone burden in the pelvis and other calyces. It should also relieve obstruction. Upper pole entry usually provides access to the majority of the collecting system and may allow complete removal of a staghorn stone through one site.[2] Calyces deemed inaccessible from the primary calyx of entry would require secondary tracts. These may be inaccessible due to acute angulation or narrow infundibula. The primary and secondary tracts should be planned at the beginning of the procedure. Fluoroscopic or ultrasound-guided punctures must be done for all these calyces and guidewires placed and secured for all these tracts. Once nephroscopy and partial stone clearance is done, subsequent fresh puncturing of the kidney for secondary tracts may become difficult as the kidney has deflated and there may be extravasation of contrast or saline on attempts to re-opacify or re-inflate the pelvicalyceal system. The main tract is initially dilated to facilitate placement of a 26 or 28 F Amplatz sheath and nephroscopy and calculus fragmentation commenced. The secondary tracts are dilated if and when necessary.

2. **Placing the guidewire:** In situations where the volume of the stone occupies the entire volume of the calyx selected to be punctured, the needle is advanced until there is the tactile sensation of the needle tip touching the hard surface of the stone. In this situation the tip of the trocar of the needle is in contact with the stone but the cannula of the needle is at a distance of 1–2 mm from the surface of the stone. It is advisable to then move the cannula on the trocar toward the stone until contact with the surface of the stone is felt. Then the trocar needle is removed and the hydrophilic guidewire is gently inserted into the narrow space between the urothelium of the calyx and the surface of the stone. Sometimes this allows the advancement of

the guidewire to the renal pelvis, but in other situations it is only possible to position the guidewire in the punctured calyx.

3. **Dilatation and placement of Amplatz sheath:** Staghorn stones generally tend to occupy more of the pelvicalyceal system as compared to solitary or low volume stones. There may not be enough space between the stone and the calyceal wall to position the dilators. This may lead to under dilatation of the tract. Excessive force to push the dilator into the system may lead to perforation of the system. Gentle and proper positioning of the Alken dilator rod in the system is important. Grating sensation of the dilator hitting the tip of the stone and efflux of retrogradely flushed saline from the outer end of dilators help confirm proper positioning in a difficult system. Lack of space makes dilatation by conical tipped Amplatz dilators difficult. The sequential metallic Allen's dilator system dilates up to its end as compared with the Amplatz dilators that do not dilate till their tip. The conical tip necessitates pushing the Amplatz dilator till the maximum diameter of the dilator is in the system. Similarly, positioning of the regular oblique edge of the Amplatz sheath inside the tightly packed system may be occasionally difficult. In such cases, placing the Amplatz sheath in a reverse manner with the straight edge inside and oblique edge outside may help.

4. **Intracorporeal lithotripsy:** The combination of pneumatic and ultrasonic energy with suction helps in clearing fragments faster, thus reducing the number of stages. Desai et al and Hofmann et al[15, 16] in their series of staghorn calculi found that the ultrasonic and pneumatic energy combination for percutaneous litholapaxy was a very effective instrument, producing smaller stone particles and thus fewer residual stone fragments after PCNL than with the

pneumatic or ultrasonic fragmentation alone. Pneumatic lithotripsy produced faster fragmentation and better clearance rates as compared to only ultrasonic energy. Simultaneous fragmentation and suction by the combination energy reduces the procedure time, intrarenal pelvic pressure and complication rates.[17]

5. **Multiple tracts:** Various studies have proved the efficacy and safety of multitract procedures as compared to single tract procedures.[15-30] The overall complete stone clearance rates range from 80 to 95% in different series. There has been no evidence to associate multitract procedures with renal insufficiency. In Singla's study, the maximal number of tracts used in a single renal unit could be up to six with acceptable morbidity.[24]

6. **Miniaturization of tracts:** Reducing the tract helps in reducing the blood loss and transfusion rate. Attempts to minimize the risk of bleeding have been addressed by limiting sheath size and dilating the secondary tracts later in the procedure only if needed. Guohua et al achieved stone clearance rates of 93% with a 3% transfusion rate by using multiple tracts dilated to 14–18 Fr.[27] Cheng et al[28] in a prospective randomized study compared miniaturized (mini) PCNL with standard PCNL for complex renal calculi (staghorn and multiple calyceal calculi). The mini PCNL group has a higher stone-free rate for multiple calyceal stones than the standard PCNL, but the two groups have a comparable rate for staghorn stones and simple renal pelvis stones. In another prospective and randomized study, mini PCNL (18 Fr) was associated with higher clearance rate, less chance need for adjunctive procedure of SWL or second-look PCNL and a similar complication rate as compared to standard PCNL for treating staghorn calculi.[29] Selecting the tract size according to the width of the infundibulum and its angle of entry into the renal pelvis helps in

preventing the overdilatation of the infundibulum and subsequent bleeding catastrophe. Use of slender nephroscopes (14 F, 18.5 F, 20 F) facilitates maneuverability inside the pelvicalyceal system to access the stone bearing calyces.[30]

7. **Use of flexible endoscope:** Preminger et al described the use of flexible ureteroscope as an adjunct to single tract PCNL for staghorn calculi.[31] The advantages were reduction in the number of tracts and morbidity. The stones in different calyces were fragmented with holmium laser or translocated into the pelvis with the help of baskets and subsequently cleared by PCNL. Combining single-tract PCNL with subsequent RIRS can be an effective strategic option for treating staghorn stones in solitary kidneys. The method gives an excellent SFR, satisfactory preservation of renal function, reduced bleeding risk and potentially less morbidity than that associated with multiple-tract PCNL.[31, 32] Staghorn calculi can be managed successfully and safely with a single upperpole percutaneous access combined with flexible nephroscopy and holmium laser.[2,33–35] Flexible nephroscopy has been of use mainly for residual stones in the inaccessible calyces with an associated large pelvis, while flexible ureteroscopy as an adjuvant was useful with a smaller pelvis.[15]

8. **Staging the procedure:** Prolonged nephroscopy time has been associated with increasing blood loss and chances of sepsis. The nephroscopy time should be restricted to less than 120 minutes and the procedure staged. Presence of infection, renal insufficiency or complications like bleeding or perforations of the pelvicalyceal system are indications of staging the procedure. A staged procedure with a nephrostomy drainage allows the infected urine to be drained reducing the chances of postoperative sepsis. It also allows the tract to mature and reduces bleeding in the subsequent stage.[36] Second-look nephroscopy is generally performed after 48 hours after confirming clear urine through the nephrostomy tube and urethral catheter, absence of fever and normal hemodynamic status.

Long-term Results

El Nahas and colleagues evaluated renal function in 70 patients who underwent preoperative and postoperative radioisotope scanning, and noted that in 91.5% cases, PCNL did not adversely affect renal function.[37] In a retrospective analysis by Akman et al, renal function was improved or maintained in almost 80% of patients with staghorn stones. Change in the eGFR between the immediate preoperative and postoperative levels predicted long-term outcome.[38] Number of tracts did not have any effect on the long-term outcome with respect to renal function.[37, 38] Stones recurred in approximately a third of patients with staghorn calculi. DM and recurrent UTIs after PCNL placed patients at higher risk for stone recurrence.

References

1. Assimos D, Krambeck A, et al. Surgical Management of Stones: American Urological Association/Endourological Society Guideline. J Urol 2016;196:1161–69.
2. Preminger GM, Assimos DG, Lingeman JE, Nakada SY, Pearle MS, Wolf JS, Jr. AUA Nephrolithiasis Guideline Panel. AUA guideline on management of staghorn calculi: Diagnosis and treatment recommendations. J Urol 2005;173:1991–2000.
3. Finch W, Johnston R, Shaida N, Winterbottom A, Wiseman O. Measuring stone volume 3D software reconstruction or an ellipsoid algebra formula? BJU Int 2013 Sep 10. doi: 10.1111/bju. 12456.
4. Li H, Chen Y, Liu C, Li B, Xu K, Bao S. Construction of a three-dimensional model of renal stones: Comprehensive planning for percutaneous nephrolithotomy and assistance in surgery. World J Urol 2013;31:1587–92.
5. Okhunov Z, Friedlander JI, George AK, Duty BD, Moreira DM, Srinivasan AK, et al. STONE. Nephrolithometry: Novel surgical classification system for kidney calculi. Urology 2013;81:1154–60.

6. Mishra S, Bhattu AS, Sabnis RB, Desai MR. Staghorn classification: Platform for morphometry assessment. Indian J Urol 2014;30:80–3.

7. Mishra SK, Sabnis RB, Desai MR. "Staghorn morphometry": A new tool for clinical classification and prediction model for PCNL monotherapy. J Endourol 2012;26:6–14.

8. Sagorika Paul. UROSCAN: Staghorn morphometry for percutaneous nephrolithotomy. Indian J Urol 2012;28:473–4.

9. Gupta M, Parkhomenko E, et al. A Multi-institutional Study of Struvite Stones: Patterns of Infection and Colonization. J Endourol 2017;31: 533–37.

10. Lojanapiwat B. Infective complication following percutaneous nephrolithotomy. Urological Science 2016;27:8–12.

11. Gutierrez J, Smith A, Geavlete P, et al. Urinary tract infections and postoperative fever in percutaneous nephrolithotomy. World J Urol 2013;31:1135–40.

12. Mariappan P, Smith G, Bariol SV, et al. Stone and pelvic urine culture and sensitivity are better than bladder urine as predictors of urosepsis following percutaneous nephrolithotomy: a prospective clinical study. J Urol 2005;173: 1610–14.

13. Healy KA, Ogan K. Pathophysiology and management of infectious staghorn calculi. Urol Clin North Am 2007;34:e363–74.

14. Grabe M, Bartoletti R, Bjerklund-Johansen TE, Çek HM, Pickard RS, Tenke P, et al. Guidelines on urological infections. Arnhem, Netherlands: European Association of Urology; 2014.

15. Desai MR, Jain P, et al. Developments in technique and technology: the effect on the results of percutaneous nephrolithotomy for staghorn calculi. BJUI 2009;104:542–48.

16. Hofmann R, Olbert P, Weber J, Wille S, Varga Z. Clinical experience with a new ultrasonic and LithoClast combination for percutaneous litholapaxy. BJU Int 2002; 90: 16–9.

17. Liang T, Zhao C, et al. Multi-tract percutaneous nephrolithotomy combined with EMS lithotripsy for bilateral complex renal stones: our experience. BMC Urology 2017;17:15.

18. Cho HJ, Lee JY, Kim SW, et al. Percutaneous nephrolithotomy for complex renal calculi: Is multi-tract approach ok? Can J Urol 2012;19(4): 6360–65.

19. Li J, Xiao B, Hu W, et al. Complication and safety of ultrasound-guided percutaneous nephrolithotomy in 8,025 cases in China. Chin Med J (Engl) 2014;127(24):4184–89.

20. Hegarty NJ, Desai MM. Percutaneous nephrolithotomy requiring multiple tracts: comparison of morbidity with single-tract procedures. J Endourol 2006;20(10):753–60.

21. Aron M, Yadav R, Goel R, et al. Multi-tract percutaneous nephrolithotomy for large complete staghorn calculi. Urol Int 2005;75(4):327–32.

22. Fei X, Li J, Song Y, et al. Single-stage multiple-tract percutaneous nephrolithotomy in the treatment of staghorn stones under total ultrasonography guidance. Urol Int 2014;93(4): 411–16.

23. Chen J, Zhou X, Chen Z, et al. Multiple-tract percutaneous nephrolithotomy assisted by LithoClast master in one session for staghorn calculi: report of 117 cases. Urolithiasis. 2014; 42(2):165–9.

24. Singla M, Srivastava A, Kapoor R, et al. Aggressive approach to staghorn calculi—safety and efficacy of multiple tracts percutaneous nephrolithotomy. Urology 2008;71(6):1039–42.

25. Ganpule AP, Mishra S, Desai MR. Multi PERC versus single PERC with flexible instrumentation for staghorn calculi. J Endourol 2009;23:1675–78.

26. Akman T, Sari E, Binbay M, et al. Comparison of outcomes after percutaneous nephrolithotomy of staghorn calculi in those with single and multiple accesses. J Endourol 2010;24:955–60.

27. Guohua, Z., Zhong, W., Li, X., et al. Minimally invasive percutaneous nephrolithotomy for staghorn calculi: a novel single session approach via multiple 14–18 Fr tracts. Surg Laparosc Endosc Percutan Tech 2007;17:124–28.

28. Cheng F, Yu W, Zhang X, et al. Minimally Invasive Tract in Percutaneous Nephrolithotomy for Renal Stones. J Endourol 2010; 24(10): 1579–82.

29. Zhong W, Zeng G, Wu W, et al. Minimally invasive percutaneous nephrolithotomy with multiple mini tracts in a single session in treating staghorn calculi Urol Res 2011; 39:117–22.

30. Manohar T, Ganpule AP, Shrivastav P, Desai M. Percutaneous nephrolithotomy for complex calyceal calculi and staghorn stones in children less than 5 years of age. J Endourol 2006;20:547–51.

31. Marguet CG, Preminger GM, et al. Simultaneous combined use of flexible ureteroscopy and percutaneous nephrolithotomy to reduce the number of access tracts in the management of complex renal calculi. BJU Int 2005;96:1097–1100.

32. Guohua Zeng, Zhijian Zhao, Wenqi Wu, Wen Zhong. Combination of debulking single-tract percutaneous nephrolithotomy followed by retrograde intrarenal surgery for staghorn stones in solitary kidneys. Scandinavian Journal of Urology 2014; 48(3): 295.

33. Williams SK, Leveillee RJ. A single percutaneous access and flexible nephroscopy is the best treatment for a full staghorn calculus. J Endourol 2008;22:1835–37.

34. Wong C, Leveillee RJ. Single upper-pole percutaneous access for treatment of or 5 cm complex branched staghorn calculi: Is shock wave lithotripsy necessary? J Endourol 2002;16: 477–81.

35. Sharma K. Percutaneous nephrolithotomy with routine flexible nephroscopy for low-density renal stones. Indian J Urol 2015;31:81–2.

36. Kukreja R, Desai M, Patel S, et al. Factors affecting blood loss during percutaneous nephrolithotomy: prospective study. J Endourol 2004;18:715–22.

37. El-Nahas AR, Eraky I, Shokeir AA, et al. Long-term results of percutaneous nephrolithotomy for treatment of staghorn stones. BJU Int 2010;108: 750.

38. Akman T, Binbay M, et al. Factors Affecting Kidney Function and Stone Recurrence Rate After Percutaneous Nephrolithotomy for Staghorn Calculi: Outcomes of a Long-term Follow up. J Urol 2012;187:1656–61.

9 PCNL in Anomalous Kidney

Rajesh Kukreja

A kidney that fails to reach its normal location in the renal fossa is defined as an ectopic kidney.[1] Such a kidney could be found in pelvic, iliac, abdominal, thoracic, and crossed sites. Renal ectopia has an average occurrence of 1 in 900 postmortem examinations. The left side is favored slightly over the right. Pelvic ectopia has been estimated to occur in 1 of 2100 to 3000 autopsies. The kidney with an anomalous position, abnormal shape, and orientation is predisposed to conditions such as hydronephrosis and calculus formation.

Anatomical Differences[1]

- The ectopic kidney is usually smaller, and because of fetal lobulations it may not conform to the usual reniform shape.
- The axis of the kidney is slightly medial or vertical, but it may be tilted as much as 90° laterally so that it lies in a true horizontal plane.
- The renal pelvis is usually anterior (instead of medial) to the parenchyma, because the kidney has incompletely rotated.
- 56% of ectopic kidneys have a hydronephrotic collecting system. Half of these cases are a result of obstruction of the ureteropelvic or the ureterovesical junction (70% and 30%, respectively), 25% from reflux grade III or greater and 25% from the malrotation alone.[2]

- A pelvic kidney lies posterior to the peritoneum, anterior to the sacrum, and caudal to the aortic bifurcation.
- The arterial and venous pattern is anomalous and the vascular pattern depends on the ultimate position of the kidney.

The potential hazards in percutaneous access in an ectopic kidney are: (1) Risk of injury to surrounding bowel during puncturing and tract dilatation, (2) abnormal vasculature resulting in bleeding from the tract, and (3) spillage of fluid into peritoneal cavity.

Laparoscopic Guided PCNL

Laparoscopy permits visual exposure of the kidney, enhancing safe puncture and correct tract placement integral to PCNL. Eshghi and coworkers were the first to report a method of PCNL in a pelvic kidney.[3] Access was obtained by a combination of retrograde nephrostomy and laparoscopic retrieval of the guidewire.

Various laparoscopic guided approaches have been described

- *Anterior transperitoneal approach:* Toth and colleagues described an antegrade transperitoneal approach for the removal of a renal pelvic calculus.[4, 5] Trendelenburg position was used to facilitate displacement

91

of bowel away from the pelvic kidney. The anterior surface of the kidney is exposed by laparoscopic mobilization of the overlapping bowels. The puncture and tract dilatation are done fluoroscopically under laparoscopic control.

- *Anterior transabdominal transmesenteric approach:* Goel et al[6] described this technique wherein the tract to the kidney is made transmesenterically between major mesenteric vessels. The benefits proposed included reduced bowel injury due to reduced bowel mobilization and manipulation. This technique is suited for patients with slender body habitus with less mesenteric fat and hence better visibility of the mesenteric vessels and a potential lower risk of vascular injury.

- *Posterior approach:* Described by Monga et al, this technique cannot be used if the pelvicalyceal system is completely overlapped by the sacrum and its alae.[7] With more medial posterior approaches adjacent to the paraspinal muscles, inadequate length of the nephroscope may inhibit intrarenal manipulation. Additionally, a more medial posterior approach that creates a tract adjacent to the paraspinal muscles and alongside the quadratus lumborum or psoas major muscles places several nerves at risk for injury. The iliohypogastric and ilioinguinal nerves lie anterior to the quadratus lumborum, the genitofemoral nerve lies anterior to the psoas major, and the femoral nerve lies lateral to the psoas major muscle.[8]

- *Extraperitoneal approach:* This was described by Troxel et al to access the lower pole calyx of a pelvic kidney.[9] Extraperitoneal access to the pelvic kidney reduces the risk of intestinal injury and leaves the peritoneal cavity intact. It has the added benefit of reduced fluid drainage compared with transperitoneal access, and may be a better procedure for patients who have had prior abdominal surgeries with resulting adhesions.

Laparoscopy as an adjunctive tool in the endoscopic treatment of difficult stones has yielded stone-free rates between 91% and 100%. Gupta et al reported a 100% stone-free rate in a cohort of four patients with pelvic kidneys who underwent laparoscopy-assisted PCNL.[10] Two of these patients had failed prior extracorporeal shock wave lithotripsy (ESWL). The mean stone size was 2.1 cm. The upper calyx was accessed in all four cases. Matlaga et al reported a series of laparoscopy-assisted PCNL in eight patients with a 100% stone-free rate.[11] These patients were left "tubeless," without external drainage nephrostomy tubes, and instead had internal DJ ureteral stent placement. D'Souza and Rai presented their data on 9 cases of laparoscopy-assisted mini PCNL (15 Fr tract) for average stone size of 18 mm in pelvic ectopic kidney. They achieved a complete clearance rate of 89% with 8 out of their 9 cases being tubeless with a DJ stent only. There were no complications in their series.[12]

Ultrasonography-guided PCNL

This technique of PCNL was described initially by Desai and Jasani.[13] It depends on the relative displacement of bowel and the kidney while making the puncture. The patient was placed in supine-oblique with a sandbag under the ipsilateral hemipelvis to move the overlying bowel away from the kidney. The operating urologist, using ultrasound guidance, makes the initial puncture. Contralateral pressure is applied to displace the kidney closer to the abdominal wall. The bowels are displaced away from the line of puncture by the pressure of the transducer probe itself. Simultaneous fluoroscopic and sonographic localization helps in selecting the lateral most calyx for puncture, giving a short, straight, and direct tract to the desired calyx. Punctures in the supine position are made through the iliac fossa considering the position of the targeted calyx. Otano N et al presented their series of 26 PCNL using ultrasound-guided puncture.[14] The stones were solitary in 15 patients (58%) and multiple in 11 patients

(42%). The mean stone size was 22 mm, including 3 staghorn calculi. Complete stone clearance was achieved in 22 (88%) of the patients. One of the patients had urine leakage after removing nephrostomy, needing postoperative DJ stenting. One patient had significant intraoperative bleeding requiring staging of the procedure and blood transfusion. No bowel injuries were identified.

Ultrasound-guided PCNL may be associated with a risk of injury to overlying collapsed bowel, which may not be adequately visible with ultrasound. Additionally, ultrasound-guided PCNL is inferior to a laparoscopy-guided PCNL in the event, a second tract is necessary. The endoscopic vision provided by laparoscopy can permit a safer transmesenteric puncture and tract dilation compared with ultrasound imaging, which provides less clarity and cannot facilitate creation of an additional tract.[8]

Sabnis and Ganesamoni described their technique of ultrasound-guided micro PERC for ectopic kidneys in 2 patients.[15] Micro PERC is a minimally invasive form of PCNL in which percutaneous renal access and stone fragmentation are achieved in a single-step using a 16 G needle. Since dilatation is not performed, potential hazards associated with it are avoided. Fluid collection is less likely during puncture and at the end of the procedure since the needle puncture site closes quickly. Both the patients had rapid post-operative recovery, probably due to lack of fluid spillage and hence no paralytic ileus.

Transgluteal PCNL

An alternative posterior approach to laparoscopic PCNL was described by Watterson et al who fluoroscopically accessed the pelvic kidney via the greater sciatic foramen.[16] After CT evaluation and analysis to optimize tract placement, fluoroscopic guidance was used to establish the tract, thereby avoiding injury to nearby bowel loops or blood vessels. Recommendation is to place the tract as close to the sacrum as possible to avoid vascular or neurologic structures.

References

1. Shapiro E, Telegrafi S. Anamolies of the upper urinary tract. Campbell-Walsh Urology, 11th edition.

2. Gleason PE, Kelalis PP, Husmann DA, et al. Hydronephrosis in renal ectopia: incidence, etiology and significance. J Urol 1994;151:1660–61.

3. Eshghi AM, Roth JS, Smith AD. Percutaneous transperitoneal approach to a pelvic kidney for endourological removal of staghorn calculus. J Urol 1985;134:525–27.

4. Toth C, Holman EE, Pasztor I, Khan M. Laparoscopically controlled and assisted percutaneous transperitoneal nephrolithotomy in a pelvic dystopic kidney. J Endourol 1993;7:303–05.

5. Holman E, Tóth C. Laparoscopically assisted percutaneous transperitoneal nephrolithotomy in pelvic dystopic kidneys: Experience in 15 successful cases. J Laparoendosc Adv Surg Tech 1998;8:431–35.

6. Goel, R., Yadav, R., Gupta, N.P., et al. Laparoscopic assisted percutaneous nephrolithotomy in ectopic kidneys: Two different techniques. Int Urol Nephrol 2006;38:75–78.

7. Monga, M., Castaneda-Zuniga, W.R., Thomas, R. Femoral neuropathy following percutaneous nephrolithotomy of a pelvic kidney. Urology 1995;45:1059–61.

8. Cinman NM, Okeke Z, Smith AD. Associated Conditions and Treatment of the Pelvic Kidney. Smith's Textbook of Endourology, Third Edition: 707–15.

9. Troxel, S.A., Low, R.K., Das, S. Extraperitoneal laparoscopic assisted percutaneous nephrolithotomy in a left pelvic kidney. J Endourol 2002;16:655–57.

10. Gupta, N.P., Mishra, S., Seth, A., et al. Percutaneous nephrolithotomy in Abnormal Kidneys: Single-Center Experience. Urology 2009;73:710–15.

11. Matlaga, B.A., Kim, S.C., Watkins, S.L., et al. Percutaneous nephrolithotomy for ectopic kidneys: Over, around or through. Urology 2006;67:513–17.

12. D'Souza N, Verma A, Rai A. Laparoscopic assisted mini percutaneous nephrolithotomy in the ectopic pelvic kidney: Outcomes with the laser dusting technique. Urol Ann 2016; 8(1): 87–90.

13. Desai MR, Jasani A. Percutaneous nephrolithotripsy in ectopic kidneys. J Endourol 2000;14:289–92.

14. Otano N, Jairath A, Mishra S, et al. Percutaneous Nephrolithotomy in Pelvic Kidneys: Is the Ultrasound-guided Puncture Safe? Urology 2015;85(1): 55–58.

15. Ganesamoni R, Sabnis RB, Mishra S, Desai MR. Micro PERC for the management of renal calculi

in pelvic ectopic kidneys. Indian J Urol 2013; 29:257–9.

16. Watterson, J.D., Cook, A., Sahajpal, R. et al. Percutaneous nephrolithotomy of a pelvic kidney: A posterior approach through the greater sciatic foramen. J Urol 2001;166:209–210.

PCNL IN HORSESHOE KIDNEY

Urolithiasis is the commonest complication related to horseshoe kidney and is estimated to occur in between 21% and 60% of cases.[1] This is likely to be a consequence of impaired urinary drainage, leading to stasis and infection predisposing to calculi formation. Percutaneous nephrolithotomy (PCNL) is often used as first-line treatment in horseshoe kidneys, especially when calculi are larger than 2 cm or after failed ESWL.[2]

Anatomical Considerations[2, 3]

- The horseshoe kidney lies lower than the normal kidney.
- The renal pelvis is ventrally orientated and in most cases, the lower poles are connected by isthmus which may be fibrous or viable renal tissue.
- The long axis of the kidney is orientated in the sagittal plane, such that the posterior calyces are orientated dorsomedially and the frontal row points dorsolaterally.
- The anteroposterior tilt of the kidney is prominent, which makes the upper pole the most superficial and posterior aspect of the horseshoe kidney. In addition, the upper pole is usually inferior to the ribs.
- Thirty percent of horseshoe kidneys have a single renal artery on either side, but the blood supply is variable with accessory vessels arising from any part of the abdominal aorta, bifurcation or iliac arteries and inserting into the renal hilum. There are no accessory vessels in the dorsal aspect of the horseshoe kidney.

Technical Considerations

1. CT should be considered for preoperative assessment of horseshoe kidneys, both to assess for the possibility of retrorenal colon and to assess the vasculature and relationship of the calyces to the anticipated puncture site. In a series of 12 patients undergoing percutaneous nephrolithotomy in horseshoe kidneys, 5 had bowel posterior to the kidney on CT.[4] Horseshoe kidneys often have extra and eccentric calyces that can be difficult to access.

2. Upper pole access is useful in horseshoe kidneys because this is the easiest calyx to enter, the puncture rarely needs to be supracostal and it provides excellent access to most of the kidney and the ureter owing to the alignment of the long axis of the moiety. Pleural injury is uncommon.

3. The posterior upper calyx is relatively easily accessible with a direct puncture in a dorsoventral direction. Tthe puncture site is more medially located in comparison to a normally orientated kidney.

4. The distance to the lower pole and ureter can be great in an obese or muscular patient, such that extra-long rigid nephroscopes or flexible nephroscopy may be necessary.[2, 3]

5. As the lower pole and pelvis are more anteriorly facing than is usual, a standard lower pole lateral entry may damage the large anterior division arteries or accessory branches from the iliac artery. Therefore, lower pole calyx puncture should be avoided.

6. Apart from several accessory vessels to the isthmus, there are no major blood vessels arising from the dorsal aspect of the kidney.[5] The risk of access-related major vascular hemorrhage is no higher than in normal kidneys.

Results: The stone-free rate post-PCNL in the treatment of renal calculi in horseshoe kidneys is similar to that in normal kidneys at 80%. The complication rates reported are also comparable with those of normal renal PCNL.[2, 3, 6–9]

References

1. Yohannes, P., Smith, A.D. The endourological management of complications associated with horseshoe kidney. J Urol 2002;168:5–8.

2. Yap WW, Wah T, Joyce AD. Management of Stones in Abnormal Situations: Horseshoe Kidney. Smith's Textbook of Endourology, Third Edition: 702–07.

3. J Stuart Wolf. Percutaneous Approaches to the Upper Urinary Tract Collecting System. Campbell-Walsh Urology, 11th edition.

4. Al-Otaibi K, Hosking DH. Percutaneous stone removal in horseshoe kidneys. J Urol 1999; 162:674–77.

5. Janetschek G., Kunzel K.H. Percutaneous nephrolithotomy in horseshoe kidneys. Applied anatomy and clinical experience. Br J Urol 1988;62:117–22.

6. Gupta N.P., Mishra S., Seth A., et al. Percutaneous nephrolithotomy in Abnormal Kidneys: Single-Center Experience. Urology 2009;73:710–15.

7. Miller NL, Matlaga BR, Handa SE, et al. The presence of horseshoe kidney does not affect the outcome of percutaneous nephrolithotomy. J Endourol 2008;22:1219–25.

8. Rana AM, Bhojwani JP. Percutaneous Nephrolithotomy in Renal Anomalies of Fusion, Ectopia, Rotation, Hypoplasia, and Pelvicalyceal Aberration: Uniformity in Heterogeneity. J Endourol 2009;23:609–14.

9. Shokeir AA, El Nahas AR, Shoma AM, Eraky I, El-Kenawy M, Mokhtar A, El-Kappany H. Percutaneous nephrolithotomy in treatment of large stones within horseshoe kidneys. Urology 2004;64:426–29.

PCNL FOR RENAL TRANSPLANT LITHIASIS

Renal transplant lithiasis represents a rather uncommon complication, but it can lead to significant morbidity and to a devastating loss of graft function if obstruction occurs. Incidence of 0.4–1% has been reported.[1] Abbot and colleagues reported retrospective records of 42,096 renal transplant recipients; based on the United States Renal Data System, indicating an incidence of 0.11% for males and 0.15% of females.[2] Buresley and coworkers retrospectively re-viewed the medical records of 646 renal transplant recipients for urologic complications. Graft lithiasis was reported with an incidence of 0.17%.[3]

PCNL in a renal transplant was first described in 1985 by Hulbert and coworkers.[4]

Technical Considerations

1. The pelvic position of the kidney and its relatively superficial location facilitate the percutaneous approach with the patient in the supine position.

2. The risk of bowel perforation must be kept under consideration. Obtaining a preoperative CT scan to exclude overlying bowel and aid in planning appropriate percutaneous access is advisable.[5–7]

3. Access to the transplanted kidney is usually gained through an anterior calyx. This is due to the anterior location of the transplanted kidney along with the change in the axis of the kidney.

4. The use of ultrasonography in addition to fluoroscopy is essential. Ultrasound guidance is recommended to aid in direct calyceal puncture and to avoid potential injury to the bowel. Percutaneous access with fluoroscopy alone is not easy, because of the difficulty in opacifying the collecting system using a retrograde approach. In the

presence of a complex anatomy around the graft, CT-guided access might be the safest modality.

5. After transplantation, perirenal reactive tissue in the form of a fibrous sheath usually develops, so that percutaneous tract dilation can be very difficult with consecutive increase of significant bleeding risk. Moreover, this perirenal fibrosis may limit the use of the rigid nephroscope, necessitating the use of a flexible instrument for the inspection of all parts of the kidney and ureter.[7]

6. The most commonly reported complications of PCNL in renal transplant recipients include sepsis, gastrointestinal bleeding, herpes esophagitis, development of cutaneous urinary fistula, perinephric urinoma after nephrostomy tube removal, and impaired wound healing and are primarily related to patient immunosuppression.[5, 8, 10]

Results: Stone-free rates have been reported to be 77 to 100% in various series.[5–11] Recently tubeless PCNL has also been described for transplanted kidney.[12]

References

1. Rhee BK, Bretan PN Jr, Stoller ML. Urolithiasis in renal and combined pancreas/renal transplant recipients. J Urol 1999; 161:1458–62.

2. Abbott KC, Schenkman N, Swanson SJ, Agodoa LY. Hospitalized nephrolithiasis after renal transplantation in the United States. Am J Transplant 2003;3:465–70.

3. Buresley S, Samhan M, Moniri S, et al. Postrenal transplantation urologic complications. Transplant Proc 2008;40:2345– 46.

4. Hulbert JC, Reddy P, Young AT, et al. The percutaneous removal of calculi from transplanted kidneys. J Urol 1985; 134:324–26.

5. Stravodimos KG, et al. Renal Transplant Lithiasis: Analysis of our Series and Review of the Literature. J Endourol 2012;26:38–44.

6. Kural AR, Obek C. Management of Stone Disease in Renal Transplant Kidneys. Smith's Textbook of Endourology, Third Edition;716–24.

7. Rifaioglu, M. M., Berger, A. D., Pengune, W., Stoller, M. L. Percutaneous management of stones in transplanted kidneys. Urology 2008;72(3):508–12.

8. Wong KA, Olsburgh J. Management of stones in renal transplant. Curr Opin Uro 2013;13:175–79.

9. Oliveira M, Branco F, Martins L, Lima E. Percutaneous nephrolithotomy in renal transplants: A safe approach with a high stone-free rate. Int Urol Nephrol 2011;43:329–35.

10. Krambeck AE, LeRoy AJ, Patterson DE, Gettman MT. Percutaneous nephrolithotomy success in the transplant kidney. J Urol 2008;180:2545–49.

11. He Z, Li X, Chen L, et al. Minimally invasive percutaneous nephrolithotomy for upper urinary tract calculi in transplanted kidneys. BJU Int 2007;99:1467–71.

12. McAlpine K, Leveridge MJ, Beiko D. Outpatient percutaneous nephrolithotomy in a renal transplant patient: World's first case. Can Urol Assoc J 2015;9(5):E324–28.

10 | PCNL for Calculi in Calyceal Diverticulum

Rajesh Kukreja

Calyceal diverticula are eventrations of the upper collecting system lying within the renal parenchyma. These nonsecretory outpouchings are lined by transitional cell epithelium and communicate with the main collecting system via a narrow channel, allowing for passive filling with urine.[1, 2] Calyceal diverticula are found in 0.21 to 0.6% of intravenous urograms (IVU) performed on adults with predominance in upper pole (upper pole calyces 48.9% of the time versus 29.7% and 21.4% in the middle and lower poles).

Calyceal diverticula are classified as type I, those communicating with a minor calyx or an infundibulum, or type II, those emanating from the renal pelvis or a major calyx. Type II diverticula are larger, tend to be symptomatic, and are located in the central part of the kidney.[3] Dretler proposed an alternative classification scheme that includes both anatomical description as well as his recommended treatment for each. In this system, a type I diverticulum has an open mouth and short neck, type II has a closed mouth and short neck, type III has a closed mouth and long neck, and type IV has an obliterated neck.[4]

Calculi occur in 9.5–50% of diverticula.[1] Although many of these cavities are asymptomatic, they can be associated with pain, hematuria, recurrent urinary tract infections (UTIs) or damage to surrounding parenchyma.[10, 12, 14, 15] Furthermore, complete obstruction of the diverticular neck can be associated with sepsis, abscess formation or hypertension. The etiology of calyceal diverticular calculi is controversial with both urinary stasis and underlying metabolic abnormalities implicated as factors.[5, 6]

PCNL for calyceal diverticular calculi achieves high stone-free (87.5–100%) and obliteration rates of the diverticular cavity (76–100%) with 90% symptomatic relief.[1, 2, 7–17] Posteriorly located diverticuli are particularly well suited for a percutaneous approach because there is usually minimal renal parenchyma between the diverticulum and renal capsule. Anteriorly located calyceal diverticula can also be managed with a percutaneous approach; however, it is often difficult to incise and dilate the diverticular neck secondary to unfavorable angles between the entry line and the neck.

Technical Difficulties

- Direct puncture is often difficult because of the small size of the cavity and the frequent occurrence of calyceal diverticula in the upper pole of the kidney.
- After successful puncture is achieved, negotiation of a guidewire into the renal pelvis is often not possible. Such a situation can occur when a stone fills a calyx so

completely that a guidewire cannot be passed through the infundibulum into the renal pelvis or in the case of severe infundibular stenosis.

Technique

A. Access to the calyceal diverticulum can be direct or indirect.
   1. *Direct:* This is the commonest access method used.
      a. Access is achieved by direct puncture of the diverticulum under fluoroscopy guidance. Ultrasound guidance is advantageous in directly puncturing the diverticulum especially in cases where the diverticular communication is attenuated and the diverticulum does not fill with retrogradely injected contrast.
      b. Once a correct puncture has been achieved, a wire is coiled within the diverticulum. It is important to ensure that not only the floppy tip of the wire but also the solid core is coiled within the diverticulum, so that sufficient stabilization is provided for proper placement of coaxial dilators. A Terumo glidewire is helpful as it may negotiate across the narrow mouth of the diverticulum into the main pelvicalyceal system giving the tract more stability for dilatation and establishing a proper communication of the diverticulum with the pelvicalyceal system. When appropriate coiling of guidewire is not possible, Srivastava and colleagues used the 'skipping technique' in which they replaced the thin hydrophilic wire with the stiff guidewire. This stiff guidewire facilitates one-stage tract dilation without the risk of bending.[8]
   2. *Indirect:* If direct puncture into the calyx fails, a neighboring calyx can be punctured and the diverticulum entered indirectly by perforating the wall of the diverticulum or by entering in a retrograde fashion, through the diverticular neck.[9] However, the indirect access technique is associated with inferior results[10] and thus should be reserved as a secondary measure.[1]

B. Establishing a wide communication with the collecting system:
   • After all stone material is extracted, the urothelium should be inspected in an effort to identify a flattened renal papilla, the presence of which indicates an obstructed hydrocalyx rather than a calyceal diverticulum.
   • Having confirmed the cavity as a diverticulum, a wire should be passed through the mouth of the diverticulum and the neck dilated or incised over the wire and stented with a nephrostomy tube.
   • Occasionally it may not be possible to negotiate the wire across the stenotic neck of the diverticulum. Retrograde instillation of methylene blue mixed with contrast may help in identifying the stenotic mouth and pass the glidewire in the correct direction.
   • If the infundibular connection cannot be found or traversed with a wire, some have advocated creation of a neoinfundibulum into the calyx or the renal pelvis.[11] Dilation of the infundibulum and creation of a neoinfundibulum have the potential to create significant bleeding. Neoinfundibulotomy should not be performed when the diverticulum is located anteriorly and normal parenchyma is traversed and dilated to form a connection to the collecting system.

C. Fulguration of the diverticular epithelium: Since the calyceal diverticulum is lined by a nonsecretory endothelium, most authors advocate fulguration at the time of PCNL. Hulbert et al, however, suggested that trauma to the wall of the diverticulum caused by the percutaneous dilation process is sufficient to ablate the diverticular lumen.[12] Conversely, others have reported that dilation or incision of the diverticular neck without fulguration results in complete ablation of the diverticulum in only 30% of cases,[13] as opposed to the 76–100% ablation rate when fulguration is performed.[10, 14, 15] The irrigant is switched to 1.5% glycine and a resectoscope with a roller ball electrode is used to fulgurate the diverticular lining. If fulguration is to be performed, the infundibulum of the diverticulum should not be dilated to maximize the chance of diverticular obliteration. Post-obliteration, a nephrostomy tube may or may not be kept.[14, 16] If ablation of the diverticular cavity is to be performed without infundibular dilation, it is imperative that infundibular stenosis is ruled out by lack of papillae visualization. If infundibular stenosis is misdiagnosed as a calyceal diverticulum and fulguration of a dilated calyx with functioning papillae is performed, urinoma with fistula formation can occur.

Comparison of Various Techniques

- Krambeck and Lingeman compared outcomes in patients undergoing fulguration alone to patients who underwent diverticular neck dilatation and found a shorter hospital stay, fewer complications, and higher stone-free rates in the first group.[15]
- Srivastava and colleagues reported their series of 44 patients. 35 (79.5%) of these underwent dilatation of the neck followed by ureteric stenting. In the remaining nine (20.5%) patients, the neck could not be localized and the walls of diverticula were fulgurated and 20 Fr nephrostomy tube was placed. Total stone clearance was obtained in 40 (90.90%) patients. At an average follow-up was 2 years, IVU showed obliteration of diverticula in 7 patients and the improved drainage in 37 patients. Two

patients developed recurrence of stone. Forty-one patients became asymptomatic, while intermittent pain persisted in three patients. Outcomes in both techniques were similar.[8]

- In an analysis of the impact of varying approaches in their series of 30 patients with long-term follow-up, Shalhav and colleagues found a 79% success rate with a direct approach versus 50% with indirect access. Incision of the diverticular neck resulted in an 83% success rate, compared with 67% success with dilatation. Management of the wall with fulguration led to complete obliteration on follow-up in 86% of their cases, whereas those cases in which the diverticula were intubated without fulguration were successful in only 50%. Overall, the authors reported obliteration in 76% of the cases with a stone-free rate of 93% over a mean objective follow-up of 21 months, and symptomatic resolution in 85% over a mean subjective follow-up of 42 months.[10]

References

1. Krambeck AE, Lingeman JE. Percutaneous Treatment of Calyceal Diverticula, Infundibular Stenosis, and Simple Renal Cysts. Smith's Textbook of Endourology, Third Edition.

2. Waingankar N, Hayek S, et al. Calyceal Diverticula: A Comprehensive Review. Rev Uro 2014;16:29–43.

3. Wulfsohn MA. Pyelocalyceal diverticula. J Urol 1980;123:1–8.

4. Dretler SP. A new useful endourologic classification of calyceal diverticula. J Endourol 1992;6(suppl):81.

5. Matlaga, B.R., Miller, N.L., Terry, C, et al. The pathogenesis of calyceal diverticular calculi. Urol Res 2007;35:35–40.

6. Hsu, T.H., Streem, S.B. Metabolic abnormalities in patients with calyceal diverticular calculi. J Urol 1998;160:1640–42.

7. Gross, A.J., Herrmann, T.R. Management of stones in calyceal diverticulum. Curr Opin Urol 2007; 17:136–40.

8. Srivastava A, Chipde SS, et al. Percutaneous management of renal calyceal diverticular stones: Ten-year experience of a tertiary care center with different techniques to deal with diverticula after stone extraction. Indian J Urol 2013;29(4):273–76.

9. Hedelin, H., Geterud, K., Grenabo, L., et al. Percutaneous surgery for stones in pyelocalyceal diverticula. Br J Urol 1988;62:206–08.

10. Shalhav AL, Soble JJ, Nakada SY, et al. Long-term outcome of calyceal diverticula following percutaneous endosurgical management. J Urol 1998;160:1635–39.

11. Auge BK, Munver R, Kourambas J, et al. Neoinfundibulotomy for the management of symptomatic calyceal diverticula. J Urol 2002; 167:1616–20.

12. Hulbert, J.C., Reddy, P.K., Hunter, D.W., Castaneda-Zuniga, W., Amplatz, K., Lange, P.H. Percutaneous techniques for the management of calyceal diverticula containing calculi. J Urol 1986;135:225–27.

13. Donnellan SM, Harewood LM, Webb DR. Percutaneous management of calyceal diverticular calculi: technique and outcome. J Endourol 1999;13:83–88.

14. Monga, M., Smith, R., Ferral, H., Thomas, R. Percutaneous ablation of calyceal diverticulum: long-term follow-up. J Urol 2000;163:28–32.

15. Krambeck AE, Lingeman JE. Percutaneous management of calyceal diverticuli. J Endourol 2009;23:1723–29.

16. Kim S.C, Kuo R.L, Tinmouth WW, Watkins S, Lingeman JE. Percutaneous nephrolithotomy for calyceal diverticular calculi: a novel single stage approach. J Urol 2005;173:1194–98.

17. Schwartz BF, Stoller ML. Percutaneous management of calyceal diverticula. Urol Clin North Am 2000;27:635–45.

11 Pediatric PCNL

Rajesh Kukreja

PCNL for nephrolithiasis in children presents a challenging scenario. Concerns that need to be addressed are:[1-3]

- High risk of stone recurrence
- Treatment must not impair the development and function of the growing kidney
- Minimise the radiation exposure
- Small-sized hypermobile kidney
- Fragile children with lower body reserves for complications like bleeding and sepsis
- Minimizing the need for re-treatment.

The first pediatric PCNL series was reported by Woodside et al in 1985.[4] Since then increasing surgical experience and improvements in instrumentation and technology have made PCNL, a standard treatment option for pediatric renal stones.

Technical modifications to reduce the morbidity and improve the success rates

1. Anesthetic and positional considerations: General anesthesia is preferred. Special care is taken to clear the urine of any infection prior to intervention. Prone position with soft bolsters below the chest and lower abdomen should be the standard practice. This patient population is susceptible to hypothermia and hence measures such as temperature monitoring, warm irrigation fluids and brief operating room time should be followed.

2. Ultrasound-guided puncture is suggested as a good alternative to fluoroscopy and carries the advantages of reducing radiation, allowing a straight peripheral calyceal puncture and preventing visceral injury.[5] A combination of ultrasound and fluoroscopy has inherent advantages over using fluoroscopy alone.

3. Staging of the procedure in selected cases, such as a non-dilated system, associated infection or large stone burden would help to decrease complications and increase the success rate of the procedure. Prolonged operating times, a large or complex stone burden along with large tract size are well established factors associated with increased the blood loss.[6-10] Kroov and other[6] proposed a two-session approach to minimise bleeding, with the initial session for establishing the percutaneous tract and a second session for calculus manipulation.

4. *Size of the tract:* The optimal size of the tract should lead to minimal parenchymal injury and blood loss, without prolonging procedural time. Tract size should be determined by stone burden and degree of pelvicalyceal dilatation. Miniaturized scopes with reduced tract size are advised as they are associated with reduced bleeding and transfusion rates. Also smaller scopes and sheaths have better maneuverability reducing the torque on the fragile

kidney and excessive angulation on the infundibula.

5. *Low pressure system:* Pediatric renal stones are more associated with infection. A low pressure system using the Amplatz sheath or any low pressure open sheath is advisable to reduce the intrarenal pelvic pressures and chances of bacteremia and sepsis. Fluid absorption does occur during PCNL and can be clinically significant in the pediatric population, with potential fluid overload and hyponatremia.[11] A low pressure, isotonic irrigation system would be beneficial to prevent these complications.

6. The placement of nephrostomy drainage tube depends upon the surgeon's choice and presence of any infection or complication like bleeding or significant perforation. When dealing with a large burden stone, a nephrostomy tube may provide access for relook second stage nephroscopy for any residual fragments.

7. Complete calculus clearance is of utmost importance in this age group due to the higher incidence of recurrence as compared to adults. Insignificant residual fragments in children are notorious for regrowth (49.8% in normal and 71.15% in anomalous kidney) in future. Most of these children will require symptomatic treatment (55.37 vs 82.69%) or re-intervention (39 vs 46%) for insignificant residual fragment.[12] In a long-term follow-up study with minimum 5 years follow-up, Lao et al found a 65% incidence of recurrence in children with abnormal anatomy and a 38% recurrence in those with normal renal anatomy.[13] Hypercalciuria and hypocitraturia were the commonest metabolic abnormalities.

Results: The stone-free rate after PCNL monotherapy in children ranges between 67 and 100%.[3] The overall stone-free rate in children was 70.1% in the PCNL CROES Global Study.[2] The method for confirming stone-free status was primarily X-ray KUB, although CT was preferred in some patients.

Results of pediatric PCNL should be further divided into three age categories based on the WHO classification: Infants (1 year), young children (2–4 years) and school-age children (5–14 years). In the CROES global study, the mean sheath size and nephrostomy tube size were larger in school-age children (5–14 years) than in the preschool children (0–4 years) (p = 0.01 and 0.002, respectively). There was a difference in the preferred methods for confirming stone-free status, with ultrasonography preferred more in preschool children. The PCNL procedure position, puncture site, dilatation method, postoperative tube application, and surgical outcomes were comparable in school- and preschool-age children.[2]

Wang et al reported their results of 247 renal units in 234 patients under the age of 3 years. All the children underwent single tract mini PNL using 12 to 16 Fr tracts. Complete clearance rates of 97.2% were reported.[14] Bilen et al in a comparative study between 26 Fr, 20 Fr and 14 Fr tract sizes noted that the transfusion rate was higher in the 26 and 20 Fr groups as compared to the 14 Fr group. Also the clearance rates were better with the mini PNL (14 Fr) tract size group sat 90%, compared to 69.5% in the 26 Fr and 80% in the 20 F group.[15] In another study by Bilen et al, the tubeless mini PCNL group had significantly shorter surgery and fluoroscopy times. Complication rates were higher and duration of hospitalization was longer in the nephrostomy group. Stone-free rates were reported as 91.6% and 78.5% in tubeless and nephrostomy groups, respectively.[16]

Desai and Kukreja in their series of pediatric patients achieved 89.8% complete clearance rate in 56 complex calculi.[7] Of these, 61% required multiple tracts and 45% were staged procedures. Findings demonstrated that the number and size of tracts were significantly associated with postoperative hemoglobin decrease (mean 1.9 g/dL) and overall transfusion rate (14%).

Yadav et al recently published their data of 660 PCNLs in 639 patients using adult sized instruments.[10] Overall success rate was 94.4%, but was lower in partial (91.4%) and complete staghorn stones (82.3%). Only 2.1% patients had complications of Clavien grade 3 or more and 6.5% required blood transfusion.

According to the CROES global data study, complications reported after PCNL include fever and blood transfusion (2–49%, 0.4–23.9%, respectively).[2] Bleeding during PCNL is comparable between children and adults.

Effect on the Growing Kidney

- Mor et al performed radioisotope scans in 10 children before and after PCNL and showed unchanged differential function and no evidence of significant scarring.[17]
- In a porcine model Traxer et al[18] found no significant difference in parenchymal scarring in between 30 Fr standard and 11 Fr mini nephrostomy tracts and, furthermore, the amount of renal scarring from percutaneous tract creation was in significant compared with overall renal volume. Mean estimated scar volume of the 30 and 11 Fr tracts was 0.29 and 0.40 cc, which translates into a mean fractional loss of parenchyma of 0.63% and 0.91%, respectively (p = not significant).[18]
- Dawaba and colleagues studied the long-term impact of PCNL on kidneys in children.[19] In a series of 65 patients with mean follow-up of 40 months, none of the kidneys had scarring on dimercapto-succinic acid renal scan. All of the kidneys except one showed improvement or stabilization of the corresponding GFR determined by diethylenetriamine penta-acetic acid renal scan.

Simultaneous Bilateral PCNL (SBPCNL)

Salah and coworkers[20] first reported the results of 13 children who underwent SBPCNL, and later Samad and associates[21] evaluated the results in children with bilateral renal stones undergoing SBPCNL. Advantages of SBPCNL reported were reduced psychological stress, one cystoscopy and anesthesia, less medication, and a shorter hospital stay and convalescence, with considerable savings in costs.

Ugras and colleagues[22] defined criteria for stopping the procedure after the first side as: Operative time >180 minutes, hemoglobin (Hb) <11 g = dL, Hb decrease >3 g = dL, pH <7.35, sodium <128 mg = ml, arterial oxygen saturation decrease >5% and systolic arterial blood pressure <100 mm Hg.

Guven et al presented their report of bilateral simultaneous PCNL in 5 patients with mean stone burden of 19 mm and mean operative time of 75 minutes and complete stone clearance in all but one renal unit.[23]

CONCLUSION

- PCNL is used currently as monotherapy and in combination with SWL (sandwich therapy) in children with stone-free rates ranging from 68 to 100%. The success rates and complications are comparable with adults.
- Relative indications for PCNL as a primary treatment modality in children include large upper tract stone burden (>1.5 cm), lower pole calculi larger than 1 cm, concurrent anatomic abnormality impairing urinary drainage and stone clearance, and known cystine or struvite composition.[24]
- A urine culture before PCNL is required, and prophylactic antibiotics 3 to 5 days before the procedure are recommended despite a negative preoperative culture to minimize bacteriuria.
- The optimal size of tract should lead to minimal parenchymal injury and blood loss, without prolonging procedural time.
- The key to success in PCNL in these small patients is staging the procedure if required, miniaturization of instruments, and using ultrasound as the method of achieving access.[25]
- The presence of residual stone fragments is associated with adverse clinical outcome and every attempt should be made to achieve a complete stone-free status.

References

1. Ganpule AP, Mishra S, Desai MR. PCNL for Pediatric Urolithiasis. Indian J Urol 2010;26:549–54.

2. Guven S, Frattini A, et al. Percutaneous nephrolithotomy in children in different age groups: data from the Clinical Research Office of the Endourological Society (CROES) Percutaneous Nephrolithotomy Global Study. BJU International 2012;111:148–56.

3. Smaldone MC, Docimo SG, Ost MC. Contemporary surgical management of paediatric urolithiasis. Urol Clin North Am 2010; 37: 253–67.

4. Woodside JR, Stevens GF, Stark GL, Borden TA, Ball WS. Percutaneous stone removal in children. J Urol 1985;134:1166–67.

5. Desai M, Ridhorkar V, Patel S, Bapat S. Paediatric percutaneous nephrolithotomy: assessing impact of technical innovations on safety and efficacy. J Endourol 1999;13:359–64.

6. Kroov, RL. Paediatric urolithiasis. Urol Clin North Am 1997;24:173–84.

7. Desai MR, Kukreja RA, Patel SH, Bapat SD. Percutaneous nephrolithotomy for complex pediatric renal calculus disease. J Endourol 2004;18:23–27.

8. Onal B, Dogan HS, Satar N, Bilen CY, Gunes A, Ozden E, Ozturk A, Demirci D, Istanbulluoglu O, Gurocak S, et al. Factors affecting complication rates of percutaneous nephrolithotomy in children: results of a multi-institutional retrospective analysis by the Turkish pediatric urology society. J Urol 2014;191:777–82.

9. Yamaguchi A, Skolarikos A, Buchholz NP, et al. Operating times and bleeding complications in percutaneous nephrolithotomy: a comparison of tract dilation methods in 5,537 patients in the Clinical Research Office of the Endourological Society Percutaneous Nephrolithotomy Global Study. J Endourol 2011;25:933–39.

10. Yadav SS, Aggarwal SP, et al. Pediatric PCNL—Experience of a tertiary care center. J Endourol. 2017;31:246–54.

11. Kukreja RA, Desai MR, Sabnis RB, Patel SH. Fluid absorption during percutaneous nephrolithotomy: Does it matter? J Endourol 2002;16:221–24.

12. Purkait B, Sinha RJ, et al. What is the fate of insignificant residual fragment following percutaneous nephrolithotomy in pediatric patients with anomalous kidney? A comparison with normal kidney. Urolithiasis 2017 https://doi.org/10.1007/s00240-017-0980-3.

13. Lao M, Kogan BA, White MD, Feustel PJ. High recurrence rate at 5-year follow-up in children after upper urinary tract stone surgery. J Urol 2014;191(2):440–44.

14. Wang F, An HQ, Li J, Tian CY, Wang YJ. Minimally invasive percutaneous nephrolithotomy in children less than three years of age: five-year experience in 234 cases. Urol Int 2014;92:433–39.

15. Bilen CY, Koçak B, Kitirci G, Ozkaya O, Sarikaya S. Percutaneous nephrolithotomy in children: lessons learned in 5 years at a single institution. J Urol 2007;177:1867–71.

16. Bilen CY, Gunay M, Ozden E, Inci K, Sarikaya S, Tekgul S. Tubeless mini percutaneous nephrolithotomy in infants and preschool children: a preliminary report. J Urol 2010;184:2498–502.

17. Mor Y, Elmasry YE, Kellet MJ, et al. The role of percutaneous nephrolithotomy in the management of pediatric renal calculi. J Urol 1997;158:1319.

18. Traxer O, Smith T G, et al. Renal Parenchymal Injury after Standard and mini PCNL. J Urol 2001:165;1693–95.

19. Dawaba MS, et al. PCNL in Children: Early and late anatomical and functional results. J Urol 2004;172:1078–81.

20. Salah MA, Tallai B, Holman E, et al. Simultaneous bilateral percutaneous nephrolithotomy in children. BJU Int 2005;95:137–39.

21. Samad L, Aquil S, Zaidi Z. Paediatric percutaneous nephrolithotomy: Setting new frontiers. BJU Int 2006;97:359–63.

22. Ugras MY, Gedik E, Gunes A, et al. Some criteria to attempt second side safely in planned bilateral simultaneous percutaneous nephrolithotomy. Urology 2008;72:996–1000.

23. Guven S, et al. Simultaneous Bilateral Percutaneous Nephrolithotomy in Children: No Need to Delay. J Endourol 2011;25:437–40.

24. Farhat WA, Kropp BP. Surgical treatment of pediatric urinary stones. AUA Update Series 2007;26(3):22–27.

25. Desai M. Treatment of Pediatric Urolithiasis: How small is "small enough"? WJU 2011;29:705–06.

12 | Miniaturization in PCNL

Rajesh Kukreja

PCNL is the standard treatment of choice for renal stones more than 20 mm and an accepted option of treatment for smaller renal stones.[1] Though associated with excellent stone clearance rates, PCNL has not been without its share of complications. Complications are generally related to the initial puncture with injury of renal blood vessels and the surrounding organs (e.g. pleura, colon, spleen, liver and lung). The most common complications include postoperative bleeding and fever.[2]

Bleeding has been the most feared and evaluated complication leading to modifications in the technique to reduce the incidence and amount of significant blood loss. The significant factors associated with hemorrhage during percutaneous renal surgery are larger sheath size, prolonged operative time, case load (center volume: Low/mid/high), greater stone burden and multiple tracts.[3, 4]

Attempts to reduce the blood loss during PCNL by reducing the tract size and hence the parenchymal and infundibular trauma gave rise to the concept of miniaturization in PCNL.

Evolution

In 1997, Helal[5] and Jackman[6] et al independently described a mini percutaneous nephrostolithotomy technique using a 15 Fr Hickman or 11 Fr peel-away vascular access sheath,

respectively with small caliber instruments. They initially applied this novel technique to pediatric population to support the smaller instrumentation better suited to the anatomy of children. Jackman et al achieved a stone-free rate of 85% in their series of 11 children with an average stone size of 1.2 cm with an average estimated blood loss of 25 cc.

Chan and Jarrett performed mini percutaneous nephrostolithotomy in an adult population with average stone size of 1.4 cm[2] using 13 Fr ureteroscopy access sheath and a 10 Fr pediatric cystoureteroscope. In a series of 17 patients they reported a stone-free rate of 94% with an estimated blood loss of 80 cc and a hospitalization of 2.3 days.[7] Similarly, Jackman et al also achieved a stone-free rate of 89% in 9 adults using this technique.[8] The peel-away sheaths were found to be too flexible and kinked easily in adult patients. The ureteroscopy sheath offering superior rigidity was then used and the length easily adjusted by cutting the sheath approximately 2 cm proximal to the skin entry site.[7] Longer operative time and the need for fragmentation of small stones as opposed to the whole-stone "grab and run" technique were the problems faced.

Jackman et al[8] defined the 'mini PERC' as a percutaneous nephrolithotomy achieved through a sheath too small to accommodate a standard rigid nephroscope. Although standard nephroscopes have shaft calibers of 24–30 F, so-called 'mini PERC' instruments have smaller dimensions ranging 10–20 Fr. A 5-fold decrease in the cross-sectional area of the access sheath (from 72 mm^2 for a 30 Fr sheath to 14 mm^2 for a 13 Fr sheath) and multiplied by the distance traversed by the sheath leads to a greatly reduced volume of displaced and compressed tissue when the smaller sheath is used. Jackman hypothesized that this may reduce the complications like bleeding, nephron damage and tract pain.[8]

Does the Tract Size Correlate with Parenchymal Loss?

Clayman et al[9] noted that dilatation of a percutaneous nephrostomy tract to 24 versus 36 Fr resulted in a comparable degree of parenchymal fibrosis. Nephrostomy tracts balloon dilated to 36 Fr resulted in a 0.16% cortical scar versus a 0.13% scar in those dilated sequentially with Amplatz dilators to 24 Fr. In a similar porcine model Traxer et al[10] also found no significant difference in parenchymal scarring in 30 Fr standard and 11 Fr mini nephrostomy tracts and, furthermore, the amount of renal scarring from percutaneous tract creation was insignificant compared with overall renal volume. Mean estimated scar volume of the 30 and 11 Fr tracts was 0.29 and 0.40 cc, which translates into a mean fractional loss of parenchyma of 0.63% and 0.91%, respectively (p = not significant).[10]

Initial Challenges to Miniaturization

- Giusti and colleagues[11] performed a retrospective comparison of standard *vs* mini PERC. They demonstrated a lower stone free rates despite longer operative times in the mini PERC group. Nevertheless, the mini PERC patients had a lower hematocrit drop in contrast to the conventional PCNL group. The most important drawback of mini PERC was the lengthy operative time.[11] The reduced sheath diameter causes a major disadvantage because irrigation

flow is limited and more extensive stone fragmentation is necessary, leading to prolonged operative time.
- Diminished intraoperative field visibility, the need for fragmentation by laser into very small stones suitable for ureteroscopic graspers and/or baskets, and the small sheath for fragment retrieval were the reasons for longer operative time and lower stone-free rates.
- Low demonstrated in an experimental study that higher intrapelvic pressures were associated with nephroscopy sheaths of smaller caliber and greater length. Intrarenal pressure ranged from 14 to 20 cm H_2O with 26 Fr sheaths but only 3 to 5 cm H_2O with 30 Fr sheaths.[12]

Overcoming the Problems

Newer design of scopes with improved vision and development of better techniques of stone fragmentation and stone retrieval has helped miniaturization in challenging standard PCNL for small- and medium-sized stones. The question of raised intrarenal pressure has also been addressed by newer open systems.

Success of miniaturized PCNL (mini PERC/ mini PCNL) in the last decade is attributed to the following technological improvisation and advantages:

1. Maintaining the intrarenal pressures below the desired limit.
2. Stone clearance rates comparable with standard PCNL.
3. Reducing the operative time by improved sheath design with improved techniques of fragmentation and retrieval of fragments
4. Improvement in stone retrieval techniques
5. Holmium laser lithotripsy
6. Tubeless procedures
7. Newer designed sheaths (Fig. 12.1) and scopes with excellent optics.

Intrarenal Pressures

- In the landmark canine study of Hinman and colleagues, pyelovenous backflow

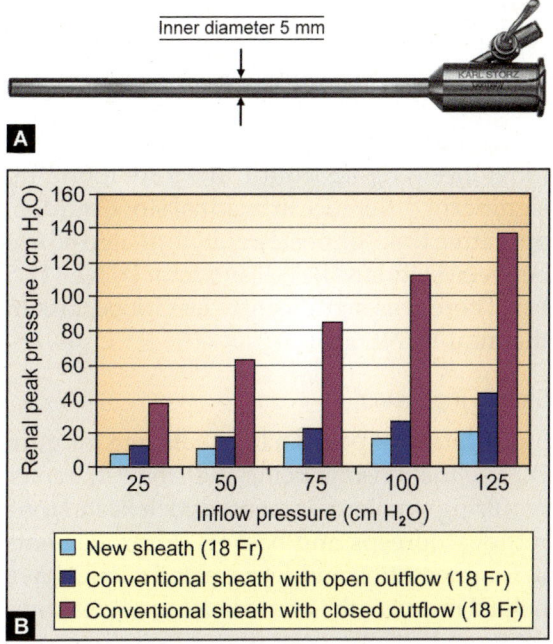

Inner diameter 5 mm

Fig. 12.1A and B: (A) The newly designed hydro-dynamic sheath with 15 Fr and 16 Fr inner and outer diameters; (B) Comparison of infrarenal pressures. Nagele Udo, et al[13]

occurred at renal pelvic pressures (RPP) above 30 to 35 mm Hg.[13] In clinical practice, maintaining an intrapelvic pressure of less than 30 mm Hg is recommended during percutaneous chemodissolution of upper tract stones, instillation of topical chemo-therapy or immunotherapy, and endoscopic lithotripsy.[14]

- Zhong et al[15] demonstrated that renal pelvic pressure generally remains lower than the backflow level (30 mm Hg) during mini PERC via a 14 to 18 Fr percutaneous tract. During mini PERC with 14, 16, 18 and double 16 Fr percutaneous tracts, the mean RPP was 24.55, 16.49, 11.22, and 6.64 mm Hg, respectively. Mean RPP >20 mm Hg (p = 0.013) and RPP >30 mm Hg for longer than 50 sec (p = 0.024) may contribute to postoperative fever.
- Nagele U, et al[16] demonstrated that by using a 12 Fr nephroscope in connection with the new open 18 F access sheath, critical renal

pressure can be avoided, even if the inflow pressure is as high as 125 cm H_2O. Additionally, a clear difference in intrarenal reflux into the collecting ducts could be demonstrated with ink-labeled irrigation fluid. With the new sheath (inflow pressure 125 cm H_2O), sections of the papillae and the cortex showed no sign of ink-marked irrigation solution in the collecting ducts, whereas in the control group (closed Luer-Lok; inflow pressure 125 cm H_2O), staining was found not only in the collecting ducts but even in the distal convoluted tubules in the cortex.

The new open sheath uses a specially designed internal channel with a curved outlet and without a sealing cap. Hydro-dynamic effects are used to evacuate fragmented stones without additional pressure or suction. Also, the end of the sheath facilitates stone extraction and insertion of the nephroscope. Complete stone removal is almost always possible without using a stone basket or forceps. The new open sheath was also associated with fewer complications arising from incorrect placement, fornix rupture, loss of access and sheath replacement.

- The ultra mini PERC has an outer (13 Fr) and inner (6 Fr) sheath. The 3.5 Fr telescope fits into the inner sheath. Saline escapes through the space between the inner sheath and the outer sheath. The ease with which saline flows out helps in maintaining low pressure in the pelvicalyceal system even when saline is flushed through the 3 Fr side port on the outer sheath.[17]

Success Rate

It is imperative that stone clearance rates are not compromised by reducing the tract size. Over the last decade, many series have now established the success of mini PCNL with stone clearance rates at par with standard PCNL.

- Mishra et al[18] and Knoll et al[19] compared mini PCNL (18 Fr) with standard PCNL

(26 Fr) for medium-sized stones in prospective studies. Both the studies demonstrated comparable stone clearance rates between the mini PCNL and standard PCNL groups. The blood loss (Hb drop), pain score (VAS score) and hospital stay in days were significantly reduced in the mini PCNL group as compared to standard PCNL. With regards the pain assessment, although mini PCNL showed advantages in terms of VAS, further studies have to evaluate whether this observation was because of the replacement of the nephrostomy by a DJ catheter or by the reduced shaft diameter of the miniaturized equipment. The incidence of tubeless procedures was higher in the mini PCNL groups.

- Cheng et al[20] in a prospective randomized study compared mini PCNL with standard PCNL for complex renal calculi (staghorn and multiple calyceal calculi). The mini PCNL group has a higher stone-free rate for multiple calyceal stones than the standard PCNL, but the two groups have a comparable rate for staghorn stones and simple renal pelvis stones. Mini PCNL has been found to be a safe and effective treatment for complex large burden renal calculi using single or multiple miniaturized tracts.[21]
- Kukreja[22] in prospective randomized study evaluated the efficiency of miniaturized PCNL against the standard PCNL for medium to larger renal stones sized between 15 and 30 mm. Mini PERC reduced the morbidity of standard PCNL in terms of reduced blood loss without compromising the stone clearance rates or the operative time.
- In a meta-analysis comparing mini PCNL to standard PCNL, blood loss and blood transfusions were significantly greater in the conventional PCNL group. Operative time was longer in mini PCNL, but overall hospital stay was shorter. Stone-free rate was similar.[23]

Operative Time

As experience increased and stone fragmentation and retrieval techniques were improved, the operative time reduced. Kukreja[22] and Lange and Gutierrez[24] in comparative studies for stones ranging from 1 to 3.5 cm found no significant difference in residual stone burden, operative time, or postoperative analgesic use between standard PCNL and mini PCNL (16.5 Fr). There was significantly less blood loss in the mini PCNL group.

Stone Retrieval

Stone retrieval posed a big challenge for mini PCNL, the reasons being the small diameter requiring smaller fragments and delicate stone retrieval forceps and baskets. Improvements in fragmentation and retrieval techniques have helped improve the immediate stone clearance rates, reduce the operative or nephroscopy time and reduce the need for delicate and fragile forceps and baskets.

1. Pulsatile low pressure perfusion pump: Zeng et al[22] used a pulsatile low-pressure perfusion pump with an 8/9.8 semi-rigid ureteroscope through a 14–20 Fr access sheath. The addition of a pulsatile perfusion pump reduced the frequency of using grasping forceps and stone baskets.

2. Nagele and colleagues demonstrated the "vacuum cleaner effect", which allows the carefully directed extraction of stone fragments without any supplementary tool.[25] The vacuum cleaner effect developed exclusively when a round-shaped nephroscope was used (Nagele Miniature Nephroscope System, Karl Storz GmbH and Co) and depended on the relation between nephroscope diameter and inner sheath diameter. The strongest effect was observed with a 12 F nephroscope and an inner sheath diameter of 15 F. It did not develop when an oval or crescent-shaped nephroscope was used. The stone has first to be disintegrated into fragments smaller than the inner diameter of the sheath. Then, the surgeon

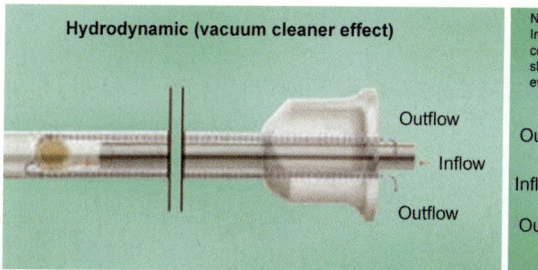
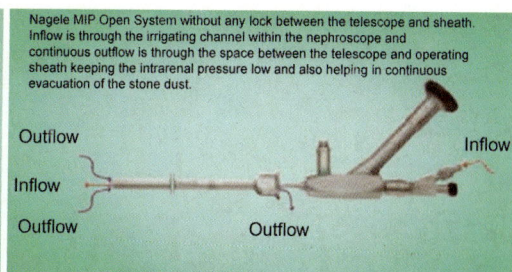

Hydrodynamic (vacuum cleaner effect)

Outflow

Inflow

Outflow

Nagele MIP Open System without any lock between the telescope and sheath. Inflow is through the irrigating channel within the nephroscope and continuous outflow is through the space between the telescope and operating sheath keeping the intrarenal pressure low and also helping in continuous evacuation of the stone dust.

Outflow

Inflow

Inflow

Outflow

Outflow

Fig. 12.2: Nagele Modular MIP System. (A) Hydrodynamic vacuum cleaner effect; (B) Open system without any lock between the telescope and the sheath. Inflow is through the irrigating channel in the telescope and outflow is through the space between the telescope and operating sheath keeping the intrarenal pressure low and also helping in continuous evacuation of the stone dust

only needs to identify a fragment, move the end of the sheath to the fragment until the mouth of the sheath is directly on the fragment, and then advance the nephroscope tip gently to the fragment. Once the fragment enters the bubble of low pressure in front of the tip, it will start to oscillate. The fragment is trapped on site and will stick to the nephroscope tip until a sudden movement occurs or the nephroscope leaves the sheath. Once a fragment is trapped, the surgeon extracts the fragment through the sheath by gently pulling the nephroscope backwards. At the distal end of the sheath, a specially designed trumpet like mouth allows optimized dropping of the fragment at the moment the pseudo-cavity collapses when leaving the surrounding sheath (Fig. 12.2). The vacuum cleaner effect removes all the fragments and also all the dust located in the area touched by the pseudocavity. The result is complete stone clearance inside the pelvicalyceal cavity, which potentially reduces the risk of recurrence of stone disease.

3. Lezrek and colleagues proposed a technique in which the nephroscope is used as a vacuum cleaner by adapting the suction tube to the nephroscope operating channel.[26] The fragments are quickly aspirated through the nephroscope working channel under direct vision. This technique helps to render a patient stone-free from even the fine sand debris. The vacuum technique is a sequence of two phases. First, it begins with a short phase of suction. Then, the suction tube is clamped to allow the expansion of the renal cavities. The alternation of these two phases leads to turbulences and swirling of stone fragments, which would be evacuated by the next phase of suction. Meanwhile, the nephroscope is moved around in the renal cavities like a vacuum cleaner.

4. Bhattu and colleagues[26] flushed out the stone fragments from the kidney by irrigation through the ureteral catheter. Remaining stones were extracted by Nitinol basket or with triflange forceps.

5. Mishra and colleagues used Lithovac™ (Swiss Lithovac, EMS) that has a 1.6 mm probe and can be passed through the miniature scopes (18 F). The variable suction energy counteracts the propulsive energy of the LithoClast. Fragments as large as 3.5 mm could be evacuated with the Lithovac™ after removing the LithoClast probe.[27]

6. Desai and Zeng[28] use a syringe to inject sterile saline solution via the side port of the outer metal sheath. During stone fragmentation, rapid removal of the endoscope out of the working sheath synchronized with the water jet period, would create a relative vacuum within the working sheath and this together with the recoil of water jets, would flush out the small stone fragment (≤3 mm) and blood clots (Fig. 12.3).

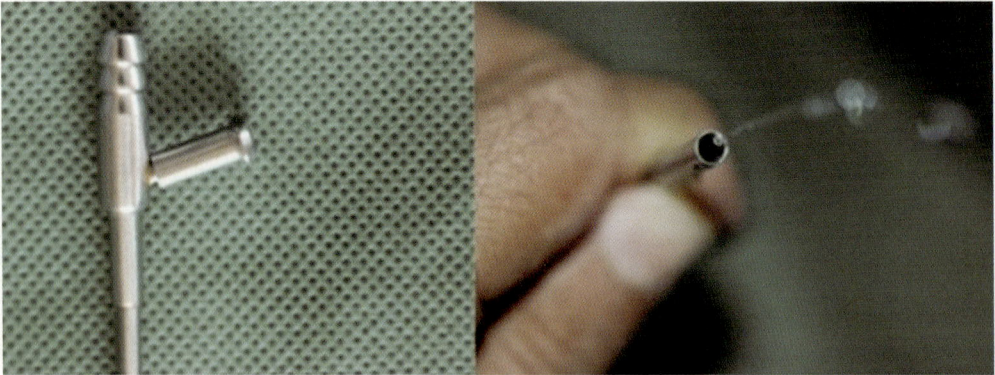

Fig. 12.3: Ultra mini PERC; outer sheath with a side port for saline flushing[17]

Intracorporeal Lithotripsy

- Reduced shaft size in mini PCNL poses a challenge for fragment retrieval. The stones need to be fragmented into much smaller particles as compared to standard PCNL. Hence, intracorporeal lithotripsy that offers more precision, control and variability in settings would be the ideal choice. The aim would be to dust the stone, prevent stone migration and reduce the need of stone retrieval devices like baskets. Smaller fragments and the dust would be easier to wash out using the vacuum cleaner effect or suction or saline irrigation.

- Ganesamoni, Sabnis and colleagues compared the stone fragmentation characteristics and outcomes of laser lithotripsy and pneumatic lithotripsy in mini PERC for renal calculi.[29] The laser fiber used was 550 μm, with energy of 0.5 to 1.5 J and frequency of 6 to 20 Hz. Laser fragmentation was started using low energy with high frequency and changed to high energy with low frequency for final fragmentation. Pneumatic lithotripsy was performed using a 1.0 mm LithoClast probe in single pulse mode. Laser lithotripsy was associated with lower stone migration and easier retrieval of the smaller fragments it produces. The need for fragment retrieval using a basket was significantly more in the pneumatic lithotripsy group. The hemoglobin drop, complication rates, auxiliary procedures,

postoperative pain, and stone clearance rates were similar between the groups. The ability to alter the settings to optimize the fragmentation and reduce migration was an important advantage of laser lithotripsy.

- Bellman and colleagues[30] compared fragment sizes obtained after different intracorporeal lithotripsy energy devices. Holmium:YAG fragments were significantly smaller than fragments from the other lithotrites for all stone compositions. There were no holmium:YAG fragments greater than 4 mm, whereas there were for the other lithotrites. Holmium:YAG had significantly greater weight of fragments less than 1 mm compared to the other lithotrites. These findings imply that fragments from holmium:YAG lithotripsy are more likely to pass without problem compared to the other lithotrites. Furthermore, the significant difference in fragment size adds evidence that holmium:YAG lithotripsy involves vaporization.

- Laser settings: Fragment size may be less related to laser lithotripter settings and more dependent on the surgical technique employed, i.e. whether the stone is repeatedly perforated, chipped, or fragmented, in comparison with worked on at the surface, by "dancing" or "painting" it with the laser.[30,31] Lowering the pulse energy or changing to long-pulse mode would decrease the retropulsion effect but would also affect ablation efficiency negatively. Pulse energy was the most important factor that determined ablation volume. At the same power levels, low frequency–high pulse energy settings were up to six times more ablative than high frequency–low pulse energy settings.[31, 32]

Tubeless Procedures

The relative lack of bleeding allows surgeons to confidently forego the nephrostomy tube. In a series of 94 patients treated with Ultra-mini PERC (UMP) for stones ranging from 1 to 2 cm, 92% were tubeless.[33] Similar results were noted by Mishra,[18] Knoll[19] and Kukreja[22] in their series as well. Tubeless procedures directly impacts length of stay, postoperative pain and ultimately patient satisfaction. Most patients who undergo UMP have a ureteral catheter that is removed at 12 to 24 hours, thus overcoming the need of an indwelling DJ stent.[33] Stents result in symptoms, health care cost, decreased quality of life and further procedure to facilitate removal. In another series of 318 mini PERCs, the VAS at 48 hours was minimum in patients with tubeless procedure with ureteral catheter drainage. It was intermediate in patients with nephrostomy drainage, and maximum in patients with the DJ stent drainage group.[27]

Armamentarium for Mini PERC
(Fig. 12.4 and Table 12.1)

- Schilling et al[34] have proposed a uniform terminology for PCNL based on the outer sheath size (XL >25 Fr; L 20 to <25 Fr; M 15 to <20 Fr; S 10 to <15 Fr and XS 5 to <10 Fr).
- The Storz mini PERC is also called Nagele modular miniature nephroscope system with automatic pressure control and is probably the commonest system used. The following table highlights the various mini PERC options available.
- Dilatation: All these sheaths have their own one step dilators. The tract should be dilated

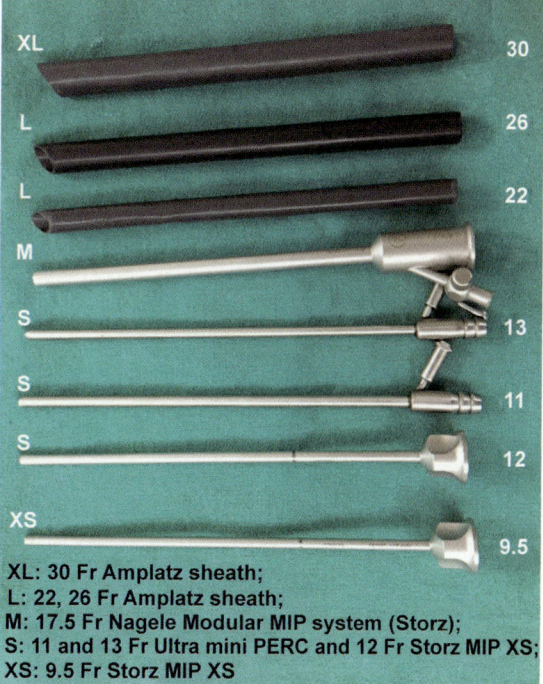

XL: 30 Fr Amplatz sheath;
L: 22, 26 Fr Amplatz sheath;
M: 17.5 Fr Nagele Modular MIP system (Storz);
S: 11 and 13 Fr Ultra mini PERC and 12 Fr Storz MIP XS;
XS: 9.5 Fr Storz MIP XS

Fig. 12.4: Miniaturization

with 8 Fr and/or 10 Fr polytetrafluoro-ethylene dilators over the guidewire. These dilators are more compliant with the path of the guidewire. Subsequent passage of the metal dilators and sheath becomes easier with reduced risk of kinking of the guidewire or loss of the tract.

- *Optics:* The nephroscope of all the systems offer excellent optics. The Storz mini PERC and MIP XS, Wolf Lamhe and the Olympus scopes have fiberoptic telescopes with excellent vision. The Ultra-mini PERC has a 3.5 Fr telescope with 17000 pixels resolution, while the micro PERC has a flexible 0.9 mm telescope with resolution up to 10,000 pixels.

- *Energy source:* As the sheath and nephroscope dimensions reduce, so does the working channel. Pneumatic probes can be used for systems offering working channel more than 3 Fr. Holmium laser is the energy source of choice for all the systems.

	Outer diameter	Nephroscope size	Working channel	Instrument size permissible	Direction of view	Length of sheath
Storz MIP Mini PERC set	15/16, 16.5/17.5, and 21/22 Fr (inner/outer diameter)	12 Fr	6.7 Fr	5 Fr	12°	18 cm
Wolf mini PERC	15 and 18 Fr	14 Fr	6 Fr	6 Fr	12°	20.5 cm
Olympus	15 Fr	11 Fr	7.5 Fr	6 Fr	7°	22 cm
Ultra-mini PCNL (UMP)	11 and 13 Fr (with 6 and 7.5 Fr inner sheaths)	3.5 Fr	7 Fr	4 Fr	0°	15 and 18 cm
Storz MIP XS	9.5 and 12 Fr	7.5 Fr	2 Fr	1.9 Fr	6°	15 and 18 cm
Micro PERC	4.8 and 8 Fr	0.9 mm	Absent			
Super PERC (Shah sheath)[35]	12,14 and 18 Fr	Compatible with Storz/Wolf and UMP nephroscope				8–22 cm

Table 12.1: Different available mini PERC systems and dimensions

MICRO PERC (Fig. 12.5)

Markus Bader and colleagues presented their work of "see-through needle" for gaining access to the collecting system.[36] The concept was based on the fact that the "see-through needle" helped the surgeon to be sure that the puncture was accurate and into the desired calyx. Once the puncture was done, the rest of the procedure was completed as a standard percutaneous procedure. Desai and colleagues further developed the concept wherein the procedure was completed through the needle itself obviating the need to dilate the tract.[37] The key component of this new technique was excellent optics. This technique was christened as "micro PERC". Theoretically, the advantage perceived was limiting and/or obviating the complications of tract dilatation.

- *The needle has three parts:* (a) The outer sheath acts as a conduit for passage of optics and energy source such as laser. (b) The central part comprises a beveled hollow needle. (c) The innermost part is a radiopaque stylet. The needle assembly in addition comprises an 8 Fr hollow sheath that can be used instead of the needle. This sheath

is useful for tackling larger stone burden. If this sheath is used, the procedure is termed "mini-micro PERC."

- *Optics:* The fiberoptic telescope (10,000 pixels) was initially used for endoscopic inspection of the lacrimal duct. The unique feature of this telescope is its flexibility. It consists of microoptics 0.9 mm in diameter with a 120° of view and resolution up to 10,000 pixels.

- *Energy source:* Laser is the choice for the disintegration of the calculus. The energy source should be set in such a way that the calculus is evaporated in dust rather than having larger fragments. The laser fiber used is 275 µm. If an 8 Fr sheath is used, an ultrasound energy source can be used.

- *Success rates:* The stone-free rate following micro PERC is reported in the range of 85–93%. Desai et al[36] reported the stone-free rate of 90%. The stone-free rate in lower calyceal calculi was 85.7%.[38] In series of 30 patients, Armagan et al[39] reported a stone-free rate of 93% in medium-sized renal calculi. In a recent comparison between micro PERC and RIRS, the stone-free rates

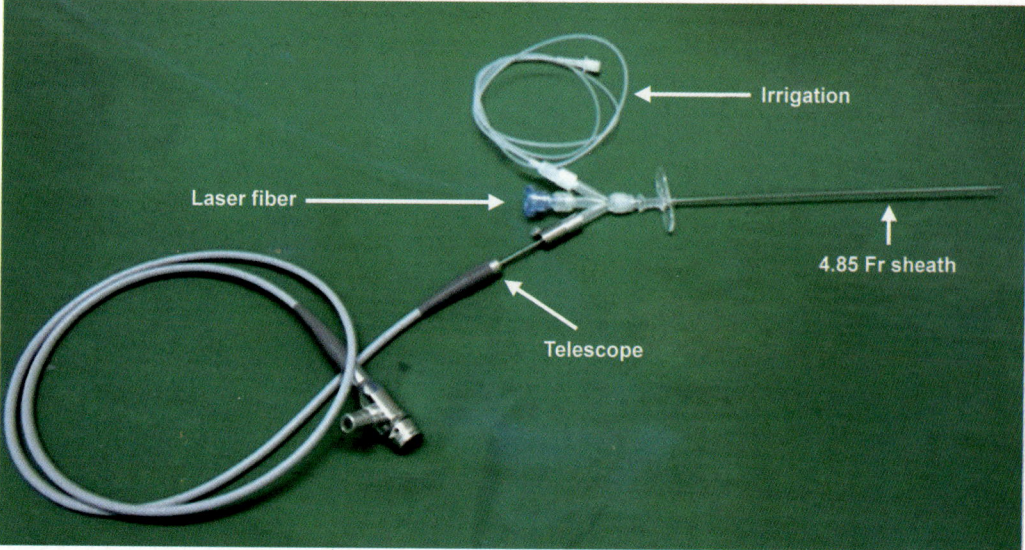

Fig. 12.5: All seeing needle assembled for stone fragmentation

in the micro PERC and RIRS groups were not statistically different (97.1 *vs* 94.1%, p = 1.0). The operating time was similar in both the groups. Complications and hospital stays were similar in either of the groups. No patient in the study in either of the group required blood transfusion. The authors concluded that, for the management of small renal calculi, micro PERC is as safe as RIRS.[40] This study suggested that the RIRS is associated with higher need for the placement of DJ stents, whereas micro PERC causes more hemoglobin drop, increased pain and higher analgesic requirements.

- *Intrarenal pressures:* Tepeler et al[41] measured intrarenal pelvic pressure during PNL procedures using 4.8 Fr nephroscopes in comparison to conventional PNL. Intrarenal pressure was significantly lower in the conventional group during all steps of the procedure. Even though there was no difference in outcome in their series, surgeons should be aware of higher pressure.
- *Indications:* Renal stones <1.5 cm especially in pediatric age group are the recommended indications.

CONCLUSION

Mini PERC has established its role in the management small and medium sizes renal stones (up to 3 cm).[22] It offers success rates comparable to standard PCNL with significantly reduced blood loss and increased incidence of tubeless procedures.[22, 33] Single step dilatation and reducing the need for stone retrieval devices are other advantages. Dusting the stones into small fragments using laser and use of vacuum cleaner effect or suction for stone retrieval, form the mainstay of achieving higher success rates. Smaller tracts may also be associated with reduced radiation exposure to the surgeon.[42] This may be due to use of one step dilatation and lower incidence of stone migration. More studies would be needed to validate this finding.

Complex situations such as diverticular stones, stones in ectopic kidneys and pediatric moderate-sized stones would be other suitable indications. The indications of these newer techniques compete with those of extracorporeal shock wave lithotripsy and flexible ureteroscopy.[43, 44] Mini PERC will not replace conventional 24 Fr to 30 Fr PCNL but simply complement it. It is not suitable for large complex stones or when there are matrix or putty stones. However, mini PERC could certainly decrease the invasiveness of multitract PCNL, in which the risk of bleeding increases significantly.

Regardless of how small the tract size is, the key to a successful procedure remains perfect percutaneous renal access. The ideal percutaneous tract should be a short, straight tract traversing the subcutaneous tissue and entering the calyx through the cup. This principle is of utmost importance in mini PCNL with smaller tracts, as an improper access tract invariably leads to troublesome ooze, which in turn obscures vision and can adversely affect the outcome.

References

1. Turk C, Knoll T, Petrik, A et al. Guidelines on Urolithiasis. European Association of Urology; 2015. http://uroweb.org/wp-content/ uploads/22-Urolithiasis_LR_full.pdf.

2. Seitz C, Desai M, Häcker A, et al. Incidence, prevention, and management of complications following percutaneous nephrolitholapaxy. Eur Urol 2012;61:146–58.

3. Yamaguchi A, Skolarikos A, Buchholz NP, et al. Operating times and bleeding complications in percutaneous nephrolithotomy: a comparison of tract dilation methods in 5,537 patients in the Clinical Research Office of the Endourological Society Percutaneous Nephrolithotomy Global Study. J Endourol 2011;25:933–39.

4. Kukreja R, Desai M, Patel S, et al. Factors affecting blood loss during percutaneous nephrolithotomy: prospective study. J Endourol 2004;18:715–22.

5. Helal M, Black T, Lockhart J, Figueroa TE. The Hickman peel-away sheath: alternative for pediatric percutaneous nephrolithotomy. J Endourol 1997;11:171–72.

6. Jackman, SV, Hedican, SP, Docimo, SG, et al. Miniaturized access for pediatric percutaneous nephrolithotomy. J Endourol 1997 suppl; 11: S133.

7. Chan DY, Jarrett TW. Mini percutaneous nephrolithotomy. J Endourol 2000;14:269.

8. Jackman SV, Docimo SG, Cadeddu JA, et al. The "mini PERC" technique: a less invasive alternative to percutaneous nephrolithotomy. World J Urol 1998;16:371.

9. Clayman RV, Elbers J, Miller RP, et al. Percutaneous nephrostomy: assessment of renal damage associated with semi-rigid (24F) and balloon (36 F) dilation. J Urol 1987;138:203.

10. Traxer O, Smith TG, et al. Renal Parenchymal Injury after Standard and mini PCNL. J Urol 2001:165;1693–95.

11. Giusti G, Piccinelli A, Taverna G, et al. mini PERC? No, thank you! Eur Urol 2007;51:810–15.

12. Low RK. Nephroscopy sheath characteristics and intrarenal pelvic pressure: Human kidney model. J Endourol 1999;13:205–08.

13. Hinman F, Redewill FH. Pyelovenous back flow. JAMA 1926;87:1287–88.

14. Landman J, Venkatesh R, Ragab M, et al. Comparison of intrarenal pressure and irrigant flow during percutaneous nephroscopy with an indwelling ureteral catheter, ureteral occlusion balloon, and ureteral access sheath. Urology 2002; 60:584–87.

15. Zhong W, Guohua Z, et al. J Endourol 2008 March;22(9):2147–51.

16. Nagele U, Horstmann M, Sievert KD, et al. A newly designed Amplatz sheath decreases intrapelvic irrigation pressure during mini percutaneous nephrolitholapaxy: An in vitro pressure-measurement and microscopic study. J Endourol 2007;21:1113–16.

17. Desai J, Solanki R. Ultra-mini percutaneous nephrolithomy (UMP): one more armamentarium. BJU Int 2013;112:1046.

18. Mishra S, Sharma R, et al. Prospective comparative study of mini PERC and standard PNL for treatment of 1 to 2 cm size renal stone. BJUI 2011;108:896–900.

19. Knoll T, Wezel F, Michel MS, et al. Do Patients Benefit from Miniaturized Tubeless Percutaneous Nephrolithotomy? A Comparative Prospective Study. J Endourol 2010; 24(7):1075–79.

20. Cheng F, Yu W, Zhang X, et al. Minimally Invasive Tract in Percutaneous Nephrolithotomy for Renal Stones. J Endourol 2010;24(10):1579–82.

21. Zeng G, et al. Minimally Invasive PCNL for simple and complex renal calyceal stones: A comparative analysis of more than 10000 cases. J Endourol 2013; 27(10):1203–08.

22. Kukreja RA. Should mini Percutaneous Nephrolithotomy (mini PERC) be the ideal tract for medium-sized renal calculi (15–30 mm)? World J

Urol 2018;36:285. https://doi.org/10.1007/s00345-017-2128-z.

23. Zhu W, Liu Y, Liu L, et al. Minimally invasive versus standard percutaneous nephrolithotomy: a meta-analysis. Urolithiasis 2015 43(6): 563–70.

24. Lange JN, Gutierrez-Aceves J, Comparative Outcomes of Conventional PCNL and Miniaturized PCNL in the Treatment of Kidney Stones: Does a Miniaturized Tract Improve Quality of Care? Urology Practice (2017), doi: 10.1016/j.urpr.2017.04.003.

25. Nicklas AP, Schilling D, Bader MJ, Herrmann TRW, Nagele U. The vacuum cleaner effect in minimally invasive percutaneous nephrolithopaxy. WJU 2015;33:1847–53.

26. Lezrek M, Qarro A, Bazine K, Najoui M, Asseban M, Benjelloun M, el Kasmaoui H, Beddouch A, Alami M. A vacuum cleaner for the pelvicalyceal system during percutaneous nephrolithotomy. J Endourol 2010;24(6):949–52.

27. Bhattu AS, Mishra S, Ganpule A, et al. Outcomes in a Large Series of mini PERCs: Analysis of Consecutive 318 Patients. J Endourol 2015;29(3):283–87.

28. Desai J, Zeng G, Zhao Z, Zhong W, Chen W, Wu W (2013). A novel technique of Ultra-mini percutaneous nephrolithotomy: introduction and an initial experience for treatment of upper urinary calculi less than 2 cm. Biomed Res Int 2013: 490793.

29. Ganesamoni R, Sabnis RB, Mishra S, Parekh N, Ganpule A, Vyas JB, Jagtap J, Desai M. Prospective Randomized Controlled Trial Comparing Laser Lithotripsy with Pneumatic Lithotripsy in mini PERC for Renal Calculi. J Endourol 2013 Dec; 27(12): 1444–49.

30. Teichman JM, Bellman GC, et al. Holmium:YAG lithotripsy yields smaller fragments than LithoClast, pulsed dye laser or electrohydraulic lithotripsy. J. Urol 1998;159(1):17–23.

31. Kronenberg P, Traxer O. In vitro fragmentation efficiency of holmium:yttrium-aluminum-garnet (YAG) laser lithotripsy: a comprehensive study encompassing different frequencies, pulse energies, total power levels and laser fibre diameters. BJU Int 2014;114(2):261–67.

32. Traxer O, Kronenberg P. Update on lasers in urology (2014): current assessment on holmium: yttrium-aluminum-garnet (Ho:YAG) laser

lithotripter settings and laser fibers. World J Urol 2015;33:463.

33. Desai J, et al. Prospective Outcomes of Ultra-mini Percutaneous Nephrolithotomy: A Consecutive Cohort Study. J Urol 2016;195:741–46.

34. Schilling D, Husch T, Bader M, et al. Nomenclature in PCNL or the Tower of Babel: a proposal for a uniform terminology. World J Urol 2015;33: 1905.

35. Shah K, Agrawal MS, Mishra DK. Super PERC: A new technique in minimally-invasive percutaneous nephrolithotomy. IJU 2017;33(1): 48–52.

36. Bader M, Christian G, Boris S, et al. The "All Seeing Needle"—an optical puncture system confirming percutaneous access in PCNL. J Urol 2010;183(4): e734.

37. Desai MR, Sharma R, Mishra S, et al. Single-step percutaneous nephrolithotomy (micro PERC): the initial clinical report. J Urol 2011;186:140–145.

38. Tepeler A, Armagan A, Sancaktutar AA, et al. The role of micro PERC in the treatment of symptomatic lower pole renal calculi. J Endourol 2013;27:13–18.

39. Armagan A, Tepeler A, Silay MS, et al. Micro percutaneous nephrolithotomy in the treatment of moderate-sized renal calculi. J Endourol 2013;27: 177–81.

40. Sabnis RB, Ganesamoni R, Doshi A, et al. Micro percutaneous nephrolithotomy (micro PERC) vs retrograde intrarenal surgery for the management of small renal calculi: a randomized controlled trial. BJU Int 2013;112(3):355–361.

41. Tepeler A, Akman T, Silay MS, et al. Comparison of intrarenal pelvic pressure during micro-percutaneous nephrolithotomy and conventional percutaneous nephrolithotomy. Urolithiasis 2014;42:275–79.

42. Desai MR, Ganpule AP. Editorial Comment: Miniaturized Percutaneous Nephrolithotomy: A Decade of Paradigm Shift in Percutaneous Renal Access. Eur Urol 297;72:236–37.

43. Ganpule AP, Bhattu AS, Desai M. PCNL in the twenty-first century: role of micro PERC, mini PERC, and Ultra-mini PERC. WJU 2015;33:235–240.

44 Ruhayel Y, Tepeler A, et al. Tract Sizes in Miniaturized Percutaneous Nephrolithotomy: A Systematic Review from the European Association of Urology. Urolithiasis Guidelines Panel. Eur Urol 2017;72:220–35.

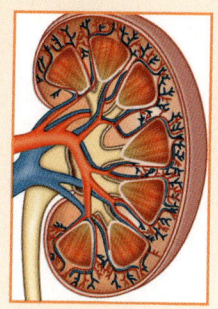

Sudharsan Balaji, Amit Bhattu

Section

II

Retrograde Intrarenal Surgery

13. Flexible Ureteroscopy

13 | Flexible Ureteroscopy

Sudharsan Balaji, Amit Bhattu

"Stay committed to your decision, but stay flexible in your approach!"

—Tony Robbins

"Flexibility is a modern day value that everyone wants. But flexibility comes with cost!"

—Maynard Webb

INTRODUCTION

First endoscopic visualization of ureter was done by Hugh Hampton Young in 1912 when he passed rigid cystoscope in dilated ureter. The first description of use of fiber optics came in 1920.[1] Concept of light passing through glass fiber was a technological revolution and gave an opportunity for birth of newer possibilities in medical diagnostic and therapeutic procedures. In 1964, Marshall reported first use of flexible ureteroscopy when he visualized middle ureteric calculus with flexible ureteroscope.[2] In 1968, Tagaki et al reported use of similar fiberoptic scope into upper collecting system through open ureterotomy.[3] Over the period of time the technological advances involved incorporation of working channel, irrigation, mechanism for active and passive deflection in flexible ureteroscopes. The ureteroscopes were made more and more slender to facilitate passage into nondilated ureters without pre-stenting. The concerns with wear and tear of fiberoptic flexible ureteroscope lead to development in the field of digital flexible ureteroscopes. It

was noted that flexion of flexible ureteroscope for removal of stone in lower calyx led to loss of fiberoptic elements. It was noted that with approximately 15.3 passes around 20 fiber optic elements were broken.[4] This leads to loss of vision gradually and need for expensive repairs. The flexible ureteroscopes were also noted to leak eventually which lead to fogging and complete loss of vision. The repaired flexible ureteroscopes had even smaller life compared to new ones. The digital uretero-scopes with chip on tip technology were innately immune to these issues. In addition to that, it provided better vision as there was no honeycomb vision 'Moria' seen in fiber-optic flexible ureteroscopes. Technological advances like robotic flexible ureteroscopy and use of disposable flexible ureteroscope are further development in this field.

With these technological advances, the indications for flexible ureteroscopy also expanded from diagnostic flexible uretero-scopy to flexible ureteroscopy for urolithiasis, for urothelial malignancy biopsy, infundibular stenosis, calyceal diverticular stones, and removal of foreign body from pelvicalyceal system and treatment of papillary necrosis.

This monogram will focus on technique of flexible ureteroscopy, troubleshooting and review of literature.

PREOPERATIVE CONSIDERATIONS

Preoperative evaluation includes CT IVP for evaluation of the pelvicalyceal anatomy. The infundibulopelvic angle and width of infundibulum of lower calyx can help in predicting whether the lower calyceal stone can be accessed with flexible ureteroscopy. Besides, the assessment of size, position in pelvicalyceal system and Hounsfield unit of stone helps in holistic planning of the RIRS. Other considerations include serum creatinine, complete hemogram, urine routine microscopy and culture sensitivity. It is necessary to ensure the sterility of urine before undertaking ureteroscopy. If urine culture shows infection then it should be treated with appropriate antibiotics prior to undertaking flexible ureteroscopy. Preoperative dose of antibiotic should be given as per local antibiotic protocols. Other evaluations required are from anesthetic perspective. Flexible ureteroscopy for renal stones and upper ureteric stone should be done under general anesthesia as it helps in controlling respiration while lasing stones, and avoid pain and patient movement which can be dangerous and traumatic to the patient and the ureteroscope respectively. However, lower ureteric diagnostic flexible ureteroscopy can be done under local anesthesia in a cooperative patient. The flexible ureteroscopy does not need cessation of anticoagulation or antiplatelet drug administration.[5] However, dilatation of ureter can lead to bleeding and it must be noted that vigorous flexible ureteroscopy with therapeutic intent in a non-dilated and non-stented ureter can lead to oozing in anticoagulated patient which may lead to poor vision. Poor vision can tempt surgeon for increasing irrigation which can lead to significant rise in intrapelvic pressure and intravasation of irrigating fluids with its resultant consequences including fluid overload, dyselectrolytemia and sepsis.

ARMAMENTARIUM FOR FLEXIBLE URETEROSCOPY

- Operating table which is suitable for fluoroscopy and cystoscopy with arrangement for drainage of fluids and allow smooth and controlled positioning.
- Fluoroscopy unit.
- Video camera and screen with recording unit.
- Cystoscope with its ancillaries, transparent lubricating jelly, floppy tip, nitinol core hydrophilic guidewire, access sheaths, flexible ureteroscope with its ancillaries.
- Irrigating pumps which can provide low pressure irrigation with normal saline.
- Ureteric catheter and DJ stents.
- Per urethral Foley's catheter.

Positioning of Patient

Patient is positioned in lithotomy position. Abduction and lowering of contralateral lower limb improves freedom of movement for surgeon.

PROCEDURE

Achieving Retrograde Ureteric Access

Cystoscopy is done with rigid or flexible cystoscope. The intended ureteric orifice is identified and cannulated with hydrophilic floppy tip guidewire. In case of difficulty in negotiating the guidewire, ureteric catheter of 5 Fr or 6 Fr size is advanced just distal to tip of wire which supports the wire and helps to negotiate the wire. Once the wire negotiates the ureteric orifice, it is advanced up to pelvicalyceal system and coiled into calyces. Then double lumen ureteric catheter is advanced over the wire and just above the vesicoureteric junction. Retrograde pyeloureterogram is done. This helps in knowing the kinks and narrowings in ureter and position of stone and mass in pelvicalyceal system. This also confirms the position of wire into pelvicalyceal system. Then another wires like Zebra™ wire (Boston Scientific—Marlborough MA), Sensor™ wire (Boston Scientific—Marlborough MA), Roadrunner™ wire (Cook Medical—Bloomington, IN) can be passed through another channel in double lumen catheter as a safety wire.

At this stage an access sheath is placed over the working wire into the lower ureter. The safety wire which is outside the access sheath is useful for stenting postoperatively and becomes invaluable in case of any ureteric injury. The advantages of putting access sheath include easier access to the upper ureter and pelvicalyceal system, multiple atraumatic passages into the pelvicalyceal system and for stone retrieval with basket. Another important use of access sheath is its role in draining the irrigation fluid continuously which keeps intrapelvic pressure low (<20 cm water with pressurized irrigation up to 200 cm water) and helps to avoid complications of raised intrapelvic pressure including fluid overload and sepsis.

SPECIFICATIONS OF AN ACCESS SHEATH

Access sheaths have an inner dilator with an outer sheath (Fig. 13.1). The dilator has a pointed conical tip with a channel for passage over guidewire. The proximal end of the dilator has a clipping mechanism to fix the dilator to the sheath. The sheath is cylindrical with a widened flange at the proximal end. The tip of the sheath has a circular radio-paque marker. The sheath is coated with a micro thin layer of hydrophilic polymer to create a low friction surface. In dual channel access sheaths (e.g. Cook Flexor DL with 3 Fr secondary channel or Aquaglide, Bard), there is a secondary channel for passage of guidewire, basket or laser fiber.

Access sheaths are available in various sizes with inner diameter ranging from 9.5 to 13 Fr, outer diameter ranging from 12 to 15 Fr and length ranging from 13 (pediatric) to 55 cm (Table 13.1). For a male patient, 45 cm length access sheath can also be used which reach up to upper ureter. The upper end of access sheath should be in the upper ureter and should not cross pelviureteric junction.

However, the flexible ureteroscopes can also be passed into the pelvicalyceal system without the access sheaths. It can be loaded over the wire and advanced into pelvicalyceal system. Wire with floppy nontraumatic tips at both the ends like Biwire (R) (Cook Medical—Bloomington, IN) are useful for this as it is less likely to cause trauma to the working channel while loading and decrease wear and tear of flexible ureteroscope.

Modern day ureteroscopes have slender and stiff tip which can negotiate the ureteric

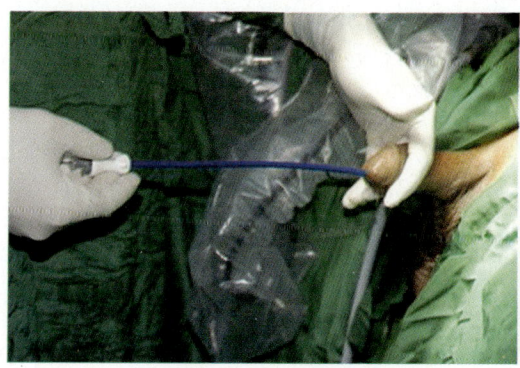
Insertion over guidewire

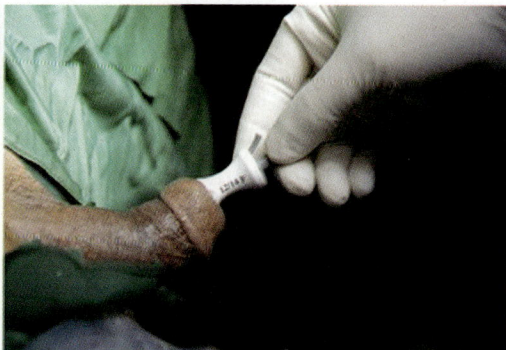
Fully placed access sheath

Fig. 13.1: Access sheath placement

Table 13.1: Access sheath specifications				
Company	Name	Inner diameter (Fr)	Outer diameter (Fr)	Length (cm)
Cook Urological	Flexor	9.5/12/14	11.5/14/16	13/20/28/35/45/55
	Flexor DL	9.5/12	11.5/14	13/20/28/35/45/55
Boston Scientific	Navigator	11/13	13/15	28/36/46
	Navigator HD	11/12/13	13/14/15	28/36/46
Applied Medical Resources	Forte	10/12/014	12/14/016	20/28/35/45/55
ACMI	ACMI-Gyrus Uropass	12	14	24/38/54
Bard	Aquaguide	12/13	14/15	25/35/45/55
Olympus	Uropass	12	14	24/28/54

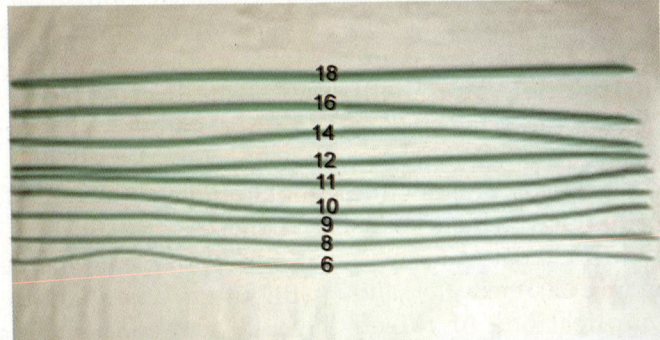

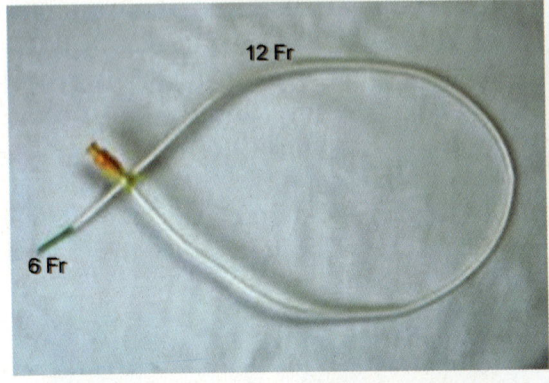

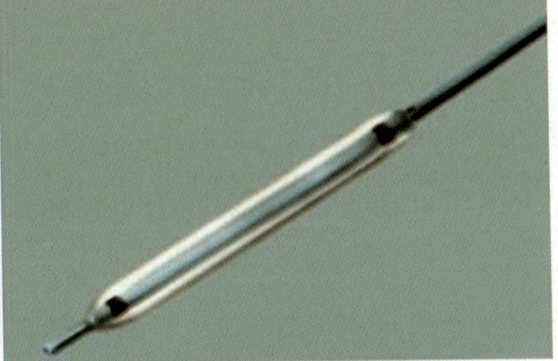

Fig. 13.2: Ureteric dilators

orifice under vision without dilatation. This does not need passage over the working wire. Failure to place the ureteroscope or access sheath in a non-dilated ureter mandates a dilatation of ureteric orifice. The ureteric dilatation can be achieved by active ureteric dilatation or passive ureteric dilatation.

Active ureteric dilatation can be done with single step Nottingham ureteric dilator, serial ureteric Teflon dilators, balloon dilator or a semirigid ureteroscope (Fig. 13.2).

- Single step Nottingham ureteric dilator (6/12 F or 6/14 F) has a long tapered tip and dilatation can be achieved with single passage of this dilator. The tip is 6 Fr and the proximal part gradually dilates up to 12 Fr or 14 Fr.

- Another option is to pass serial Teflon ureteric dilators. These consist of multiple ureteric dilators of serially increasing diameters (6, 8, 9, 10, 11, 12, 14, 16, 18 Fr) which need to be passed over the working wire one after the other (Fig. 13.3).
- Active dilatation can also be achieved with ureteric balloon dilators. Balloon of the balloon dilator is around 4–6 cm in length and the diameter of balloon is 4–6 mm on inflation. In collapsed state the diameter is 3–7 Fr varying as per the make (passport/ascend). The balloon dilator has markings at the proximal end and distal end of balloon which assists its placement at the ureteric orifice or any other narrowing in ureter under fluoroscopic control. Then the balloon is inflated with mildly diluted contrast till the waisting at tight portion disappears on fluoroscopic control. Generally dilatation up to 4 mm diameter (12 Fr) is sufficient.
- Another way for dilatation of ureter is to pass the semirigid ureteroscope under vision into lower ureter. The passage of semirigid ureteroscope through vesicoureteric junction into lower ureter leads to dilatation to admit flexible ureteroscope or access sheath. Then either the flexible ureteroscope is passed over wire or directly or access sheath is placed into lower ureter over wire.

If despite this gentle maneuvering the ureteroscope cannot be passed or access sheath cannot be placed, then it is advisable to stage procedure by placing DJ stent. DJ stent achieves passive dilatation of ureter over 7–14 days. This not only avoids trauma to ureter but also helps in allowing easy passage of access sheath and/or ureteroscope after 7–14 days. This dilated ureter also allows maintaining lower intra-pelvic pressure during later procedure.

FLEXIBLE URETEROSCOPES

It can be a fiberoptic (conventional) or digital (chip on tip) ureteroscopes depending on the way, the image is carried from the tip to the control of body (Fig. 13.4). The basic design consists of a control body, shaft and tip of the ureteroscope.

Fiberoptic Ureteroscopes

The control body of the scope remains outside the patient and acts as a handle for the surgeon. It has the deflecting controls, working channel, irrigation channel, light post, eyepiece with focussing component and a vent port (Fig. 13.5). All the currently

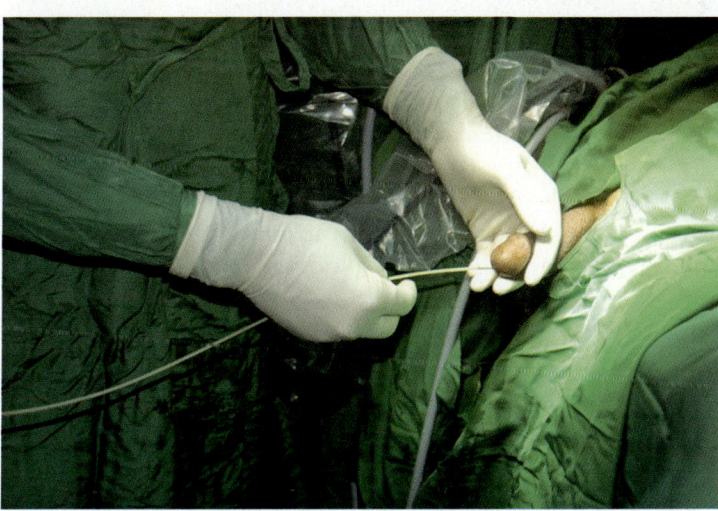

Fig. 13.3: Serial ureteric dilation

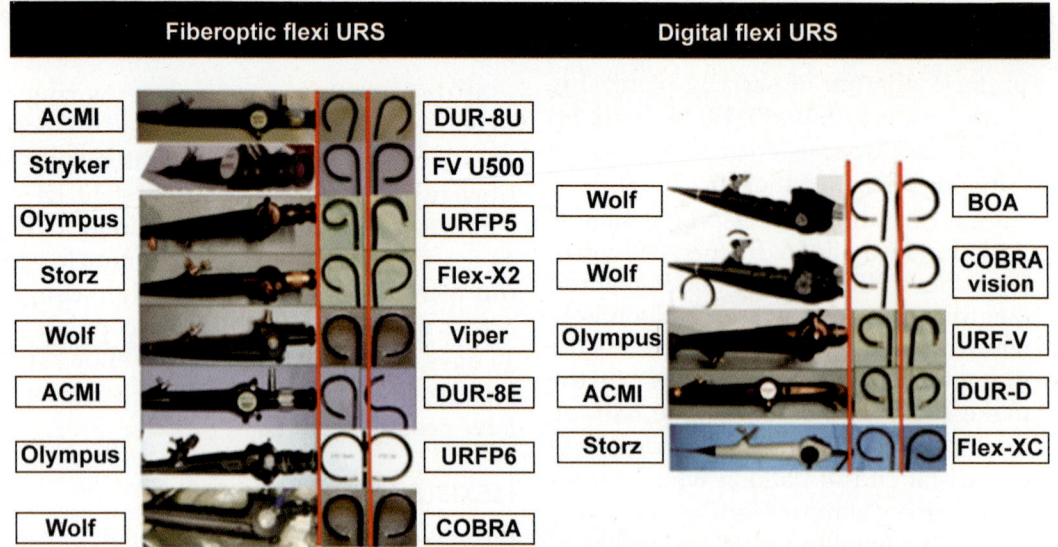

Fig. 13.4: Various flexible ureteroscopes (*Courtesy*: Dr Olivier Traxer, Paris, France)

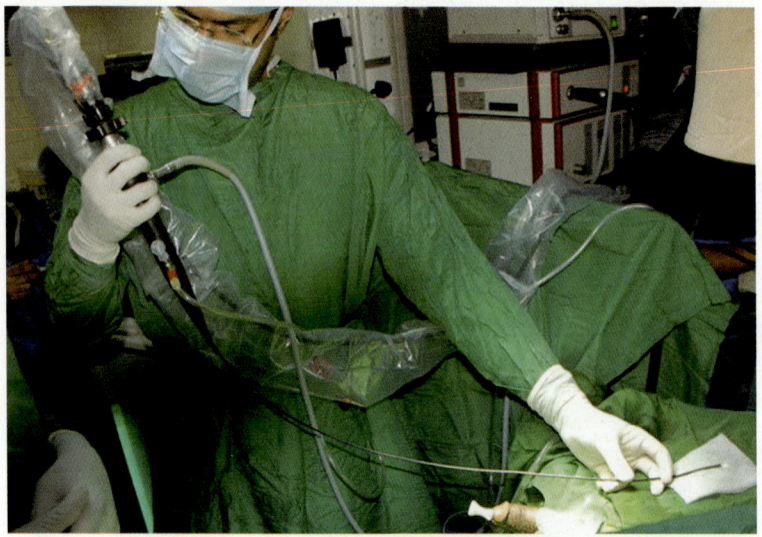

Fig. 13.5: Fully assembled ureteroscope

available fiberoptic ureteroscopes have a working channel of 3.6 Fr permitting the use of instruments up to 3 Fr along with irrigation, except the dual channel Wolf COBRA (3.3 Fr × 2) ureteroscope. The irrigation port is connected to the working channel at right angle. The eyepiece magnifies the virtual image and focussing component is available.

The shaft encloses the fiberoptic bundles which are coherent and non-coherent for transmission of image and light respectively, working channel (3.6 Fr) and wires for deflection mechanism. There are minor variations with the diameter of tip and shaft and the working length according to the manufacturer are listed in Table 13.2.

The objective end contains 2–9 lenses for conversion of the light into an image and the angle of view is 0°. There is an added prism if the ureteroscope provides different viewing

Table 13.2: List of fiberoptic ureteroscopes

Ureteroscope	Working channel (Fr)	Max deflection (up/down)	Tip diameter (Fr)	Shaft diameter (Fr)	Working length (cm)	Angle of view
Flex-X2 (Storz)	3.6	270/270	7.5	8.4	64	0°
Viper (Wolf)	3.6	270/270	6	8.8	68	0°
COBRA (Wolf)	2 × 3.3	270/270	6	9.9	68	0°
DUR 8 Elite (ACMI)	3.6	1° (170/180) 2° (130)	6.75	8.6	64	9°
URFP5 (Olympus)	3.6	180/275	5.3	7.95	70	0°
URFP6 (Olympus)	3.6	275/275	4.9	7.95	64	0°

angles. The distal end of the working channel opens below the fiberoptic bundles. The distal end of the working channel has a ceramic (Laserite™) coating for 1.5 cm to prevent any thermal injury. Field of view and the deflection of all the commonly available ureteroscopes are enlisted in Table 13.2.

DIGITAL URETEROSCOPES (Table 13.3)

The body has a working channel, irrigation channel and deflecting lever. There is no ocular lens or a focussing component in a digital ureteroscope and there is no need to attach the camera head making it lighter to handle.

In a digital ureteroscope, the image is captured by a camera located at the tip of the ureteroscope and the image is converted to electrical signals by the video chip. Two types of imaging chips are used in digital scopes, viz. complementary metal oxide semiconductor (CMOS) and charged coupled device (CCD). In a CMOS sensor, the chip gives output as digital bits as each pixel converts the charge to voltage, and the sensor in itself has amplifiers, noise correction, and digitization circuits. Although the CMOS imagers require less energy, process images faster, run at cooler temperatures, compact and less expensive, the design has inherent disadvantages of increased complexity, lesser available area for light capture and a lower uniformity due to individual conversions. In a CCD sensor, every pixel's charge is transferred through output nodes and converted to voltage, buffered, and sent as an analog signal.

Table 13.3: List of digital ureteroscopes

Ureteroscope	Working channel (Fr)	Max deflection (up/down)	Tip diameter (Fr)	Shaft diameter (Fr)	Working length (cm)	Angle of view	Field of view	Chip technology
Flex-Xc (Storz)	3.6	270/270	8.4	8.5	70	0°	90	CMOS
URF-V (Olympus)	3.6	180/275	8.5	9.9	67	0°	90	CCD
URFV2 (Olympus)	3.6	275/275	8.5	8.4	64	0°	90	CCD
BOA (Wolf)	3.6	270/270	6.6	8.7	67	0°	90	CMOS
COBRA (Wolf)	2.4/3.6	270/270	5.5	9.9	67	0°	90	CMOS
Invisio D-URD	3.6	250/250	8.7	9.3	65	0°	80	CMOS

In comparison, CCD imagers are a mature technology that has high sensitivity and is less affected by signal noise, all of the pixel can be devoted to light capture, and hence the output's uniformity is high. Overall, as the chip at the tip receives the image directly, the pixel resolution is nearly ten times that of fiberoptic ureteroscopes.

Thus, there are no coherent fiber bundles (as there is no necessity for image transmission) and the non-coherent bundle transfers the light through the shaft. In a few scopes, the light bundles are divided into two, one on either side of the objective lens providing a more uniform lighting than the fiberoptic ureteroscopes.

Manipulation of the Ureteroscope

The flexible ureteroscope is held so that the channel for accessories is easily accessible. The surgeon holds the ureteroscope with the dominant hand, with the thumb on the deflection lever. The other hand stabilizes the shaft at the meatus (Fig. 13.6). The assistant is responsible for maintaining irrigation and passing the accessories without obstructing the movements of the surgeon. There are 3 possible movements with the ureteroscope, namely right-left rotation (horizontal, X axis), up-down deflection (vertical, Y axis) and push-remove (depth, Z axis) (Fig. 13.7).

When dealing with the right kidney, the calyces lie on the left side of the viewing screen and the dominant hand needs to be supinated to rotate the scope. For the left kidney, the calyces lie on the right side of the screen and the dominant hand needs to be pronated to rotate the scope towards the calyces. Deflection requires movement of the deflecting lever on the control of body (Figs 13.8 and 13.9). The ureteroscopes can be intuitive (logic, positive, American) if the direction of the tip of the lever corresponds to that of the scope tip, i.e. up is up and down is down. Counter-intuitive (antilogic, negative, European) scopes have opposing movements between the scope tip and the deflecting lever, i.e. up is down and down is up. Active deflection refers to the deflection of the control lever resulting in the deflection of the tip of

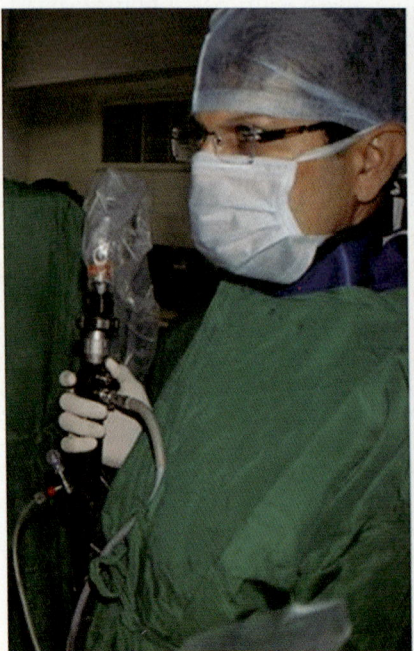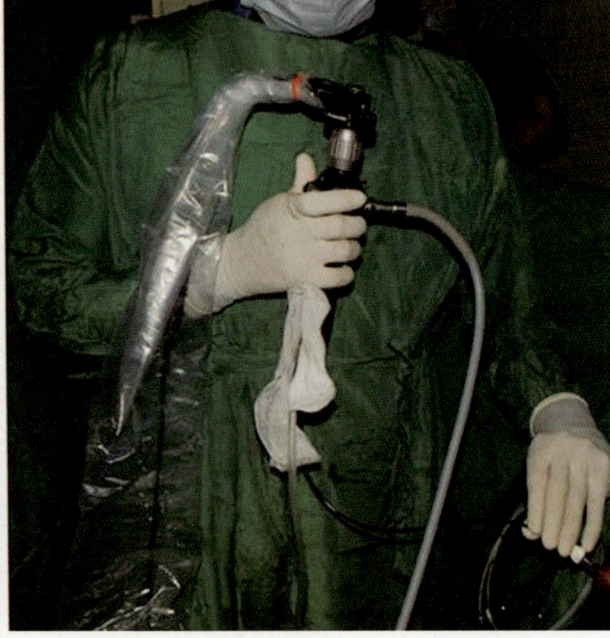

Fig. 13.6: Proper holding of the ureteroscope

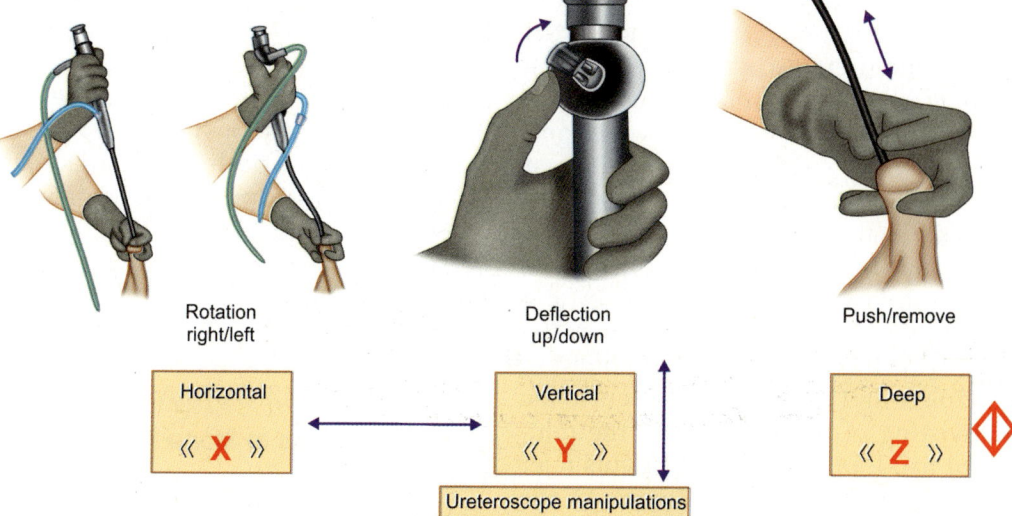

Rotation right/left

Deflection up/down

Push/remove

Horizontal	Vertical	Deep
« X »	« Y »	« Z »

Ureteroscope manipulations

Fig. 13.7: Ureteroscope manipulation in 3 different axes

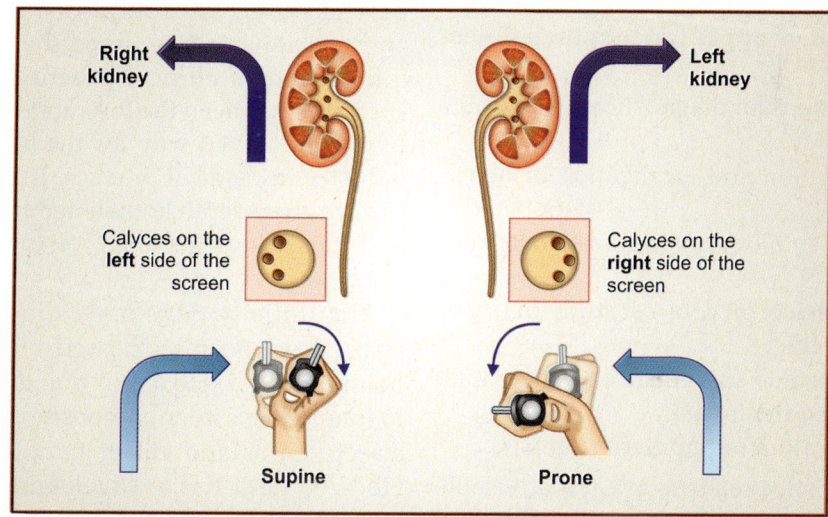

Fig. 13.8: Summary of dominant hand movements (*Courtesy*: Dr Olivier Traxer, Paris, France)

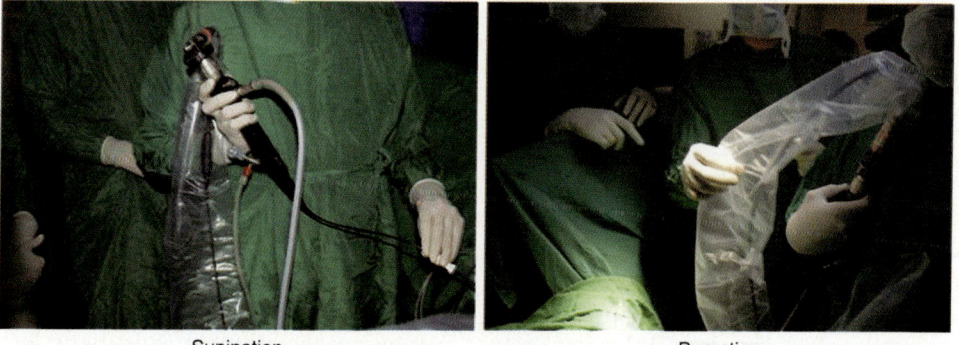

Supination

Pronation

Fig. 13.9: Supination and pronation

ureteroscope through the wires along the shaft. Passive deflection refers to exaggerated bending of the ureteroscope tip by bending the shaft against the wall of the renal pelvis. Deflection of all available ureteroscopes gets reduced with the passing of laser fiber or baskets corresponding to the size of the passed ancillaries. Dual deflection systems of the yester-generation scopes are no longer required with this improved technology and slender scopes. Macrorotation refers to the movement of the dominant hand holding the handpiece and microrotation refers to the slight twisting of the shaft using the non-dominant hand. In and out movements refer to the push or retracting movements of the ureteroscope using the non-dominant hand.

Diagnostic applications of flexible ureteroscopy and treatment of upper tract urothelial neoplasia

The indications for diagnostic use of flexible ureteroscopy are:

- Investigation and localization of hematuria
- Positive cytology not localized to urinary bladder
- Filling defect on contrast study of upper urinary tract
- Resection and surveillance of upper tract urothelial malignancy
- Identification of papillary necrosis

For diagnostic ureteroscopy, it is advisable to first do the ureteroscopy with semirigid ureteroscope passed across ureteric orifice into ureter without wire. This prevents the artefacts created by passage of wire over the ureteric mucosa. Semirigid ureteroscope is passed up the ureter as high as possible to assess the ureteric mucosa for any lesion. If any lesion is present it is biopsied. After this the wire is passed through the semirigid ureteroscope into the pelvicalyceal system. It is parked with its tip into pelvicalyceal system. The flexible ureteroscope is passed directly into the ureter across the ureteric orifice over the wire or it is passed through the ureteric

access sheath. The upper ureter and pelvicalyceal system is carefully examined with flexible ureteroscope. After this the suspicious lesion is biopsied. The options of devices for biopsies are cup biopsy forceps, BIGopsy® forceps (Cook Medical—Bloomington, IN). If multiple lesions are present and representative biopsies are taken, the rest of the lesions may be fulgurated with Ho:YAG laser or with Bugbee™ electrode.

FLEXIBLE URETERORENOSCOPY FOR TREATMENT OF UROLITHIASIS

FURS and Lasers in Stone Management

Lasers and FURS go hand in hand in current day urological practice. Intra-corporeal electrohydraulic lithotripters are a thing of the past and lasers have surpassed in both usage and efficiency. Ever since the lasers were introduced in clinical practice, urological speciality has been the foremost to utilize and ultimately paved way for the booming laser industry in medical practice. It is imperative to have an in-depth knowledge about the laser and its settings for a successful FURS for a calculus.

The initially developed diode and ruby lasers have been surpassed by the current holmium laser (Ho:YAG) due to their ability to fragment all stone compositions, better cost effectiveness and easier maintenance. The Ho:YAG laser has a wavelength of 2100 nm and is absorbed within 3 mm of the surrounding water and is very safe for intracorporeal lithotripsy and practically causes no damage to the urothelium, unless upon direct contact activation. Ho:YAG causes stone fragmentation by photothermal mechanisms: Direct light absorption by the stone surfaces creating a very high temperature of the stones and subsequent thermal breakdown. This has been confirmed with the observation of "glowing hot fragments" with synchronized photography. Further, activation of laser causes vaporization of fluid between the tip of laser fiber and the stone resulting in more direct energy transfer (Moses effect).[6] The same photothermal processes are found responsible for the finer fragments obtained with Ho:YAG laser lithotripsy. Thulium fiber laser (TFL) and erbium:YAG are currently being investigated as an equivalent or better alternatives to Ho:YAG laser. These are still in elementary stages due to lack of proper and durable laser fiber issues.

Ho:YAG laser utilizes quartz fiber which is both reusable and flexible. A laser fiber has a central quartz (silica) core which is surrounded by 'cladding' and both these together constitute the 'optical core' (Fig. 13.10). The optical core is surrounded by a plastic coating and this end firing laser fiber is used for stone fragmentation. Conflicting reports have been published regarding the effect of increasing laser fiber diameter (200, 273, 365, 550 microns) and lithotripsy performance. Larger diameter fibers produce a wider ablation fissure whereas, the smaller fibers act as a fine drill, producing a narrow and deep ablation as the energy is concentrated on the tip of laser fiber. In clinical practice, best results have been obtained with the 273 and 365 micron fibers as the smaller fibers core through the stone leading to premature stone fragmentation resulting in multiple fragments and the larger fibers may not have sufficient energy at the tip, especially with lower energy settings as the energy gets dispersed throughout the

entire surface of the laser fiber tip and does not exceed the ablation threshold. Other disadvantages of larger laser fibers include impaired deflection of the ureteroscope, decreased water inflow and poor vision and stone retropulsion. Recent studies have created serious doubts on the manufacturer's credibility as similar sized laser fibers from different companies did not meet the specified size. It is imperative to sort the issue at the earliest to avoid any adverse impact on the patient or the ureteroscope.

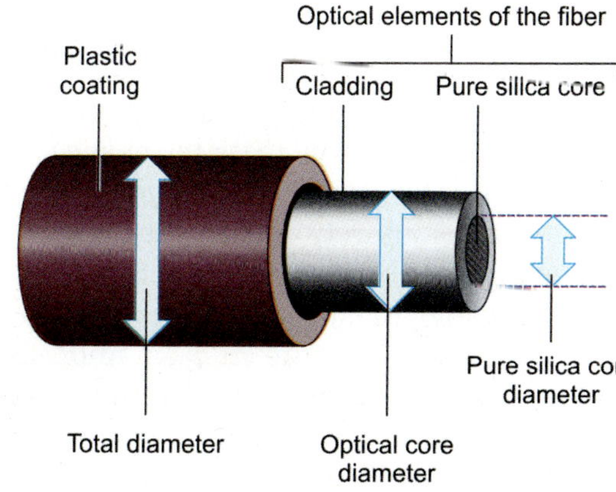

With continued laser emission, the fiber tip wears off and degrades by "Burn back effect". High pulse energy, smaller fiber diameter and short pulse mode increase the fiber tip degradation by concentrating the energy at the tip. Hard stones also promote fiber degradation by more opacification and burn back effect. Once the fiber tip degrades, the current practice to freshen the tip with suture cutting scissors is found to decrease the efficiency of the laser fiber. Even when using a new fiber, stripping the laser fiber tip reduces the efficiency and is no longer advocated.

Laser energy is the amount of energy that is delivered at the tip of laser fiber and frequency is the speed at which it is delivered. Total power of the laser is the product of pulse energy (joules) and frequency (hertz). For a fixed power output from the laser fiber, increasing energy causes more stone ablation, whereas the same is not true when increasing the pulse frequency. High power with low frequency was found to be six times more efficient in stone ablation compared to low power with high frequency (Table 13.4).

Other new advances in laser delivery systems are the introduction of adjustment in pulse duration. In short pulse and long pulse modes, the energy is delivered for 180–330 µs and 650–1200 µs, respectively. The entire energy is concentrated at the laser tip for a short period of time in a short pulse and hence the short pulse mode is more efficient for stone

Fig. 13.10: Laser fiber

Table 13.4: Laser settings during FURS (generalized)		
Technique	Energy (J)	Frequency (Hz)
Dusting	Low energy (0.2–0.5)	High frequency (15–60)
Basketing	High energy (0.6–2.0)	Low frequency (4–6)
Popcornig	Moderate energy (1.0)	Moderate frequency (10–15)

ablation (25% more than the long pulse mode). In the long pulse mode, the energy is distributed over a long period of time and hence the peak energy at any given point of time is less at the laser tip. This is found true across all laser settings. The disadvantage of increasing the pulse energy and short pulse modes are the increased retropulsion.

Regarding the size of the fragments after laser lithotripsy, usage of low energy and high frequency is claimed to dust the stone, whereas high energy with low frequency causes stone fragmentation. In a series of experiments using automated laser delivery systems, this traditional view has been questioned. Even if the laser settings affect the fragment size, the effect is second to the surgical technique only. To dust the stone, the stone should be "painted" and the laser fiber should be "dancing" on the stone surface. "Coring in" to the stone results in fragmentation and increased fragment size irrespective of the laser settings. A practical guide to the laser settings are given below for achieving the best possible effect.

A. Management of Upper Ureteric Stones

Management of upper ureteric stone requires use of flexible ureteroscope due to natural lie of upper ureter. In most patients, upper ureter allows the introduction of semirigid ureteroscope but achieving lithotripsy in upper ureter is difficult. A semirigid ureteroscope in upper ureter naturally shows the anterior wall of upper ureter due to passage over bony pelvis in middle ureter and the stones fall back on the dependent posterior wall in supine patients.

The preferred position of treatment of an upper ureteric stone is lithotomy with mild Trendelenburg position. For flexible ureteroscopy the access to upper ureter is achieved as described above. It is preferable to pass the wire across the stone into the PCS. This wire placement may be impossible to achieve in case of an impacted ureteric calculus wherein the wire is placed up to the stone. If access sheath is used it is placed up to the midureter only. If access sheath is not put it is advisable to put small infant feeding tube (6 Fr) to drain the bladder and prevent rise in bladder pressure which will eventually lead to poor vision due to poor ureteric drainage. Stones in upper ureter are dusted with laser settings of higher frequency (15–20 Hz) and lower energy (0.6–1 J). This setting allows it to be completely dusted and there is no need to retrieve any fragment.

Different techniques are available to prevent the stone migration into the PCS. The regular use of holmium laser lithotripsy has considerable reduced the stone retropulsion. It is also advantageous to use thinner optical fibers (200 μm or 273 μm) to avoid stone migration. Further, the use of short laser pulse duration at full width and maximum height, higher energies regardless of pulse duration and larger laser fibers increase the chances of retropulsion. This can be further minimized with the use of antiretropulsion devices or a combination of lithotripsy with suction. Stone Cone™ (Boston Scientific, USA) is a nitinol device with a shaft size of 3 Fr and can conform into a cone of size 7–10 mm when deployed beyond the stone. NTrap™ (Cook Medical, Spencer, IN) has a shaft size of 2.8 Fr and has an expandable umbrella of size 7 mm to prevent the stone from getting pushed up. CoAx™ Stone Control Device (Accordion Medical, PercSys, USA) has a polyurethane film which conforms to the shape of the ureter and prevents migration. Instillation of lignocaine jelly has also been advocated to occlude the ureter above the stone by few authors. BackStop® (Boston Scientific, USA) is a thermosensitive polymer which when injected forms a gel at body temperature and prevents stone retropulsion, and can be flushed after completion of procedure by injecting cold saline. Although the immediate cost of ureteroscopy is increased with these devices, cost effectiveness is achieved by reducing the operating room time and cost and need for auxiliary retrieval devices and procedures.

Despite these maneuvers, quite often the stone will disimpact and fragments will migrate up to the pelvicalyceal system. These fragments may be basketted with nitinol baskets or the fragments can be further dusted to passable dust. The advantage of retrieval of fragments with basket is that it allows for chemical analysis of stones which can be directed towards measures to prevent recurrence of stones.

It is not always necessary to put a DJ stent in patients with dilated ureter and patient who were pre-stented. It is advisable to review the ureter at end of the flexible ureteroscopy particularly when access sheath is used for any ureteric injury. In case of any injury it is advisable to stent the ureter. The indication of putting stent post-operatively are tight ureter, suspected ureteric injury, prolonged procedures, large volume of stone fragments, suspicion of infection or infective stone. Even though the stent may give rise to lower urinary tract symptoms, it definitely improves the passage of stone fragments and minimizes need for emergency colic visit due to passage of fragments.

B. Management of Small Renal Stones (Middle Calyx and Upper Calyx)

This is one of the most common indications for RIRS. The stones in the middle calyx and upper calyx can be treated *in situ* with flexible ureteroscopy. Stones may be lased with Ho: YAG laser with either fragmentation or dusting setting. The fragments when sufficiently small can be taken out with basket. An access sheath specifically suits this need for multiple passes for retrieval of stone fragments. A 12 Fr inner diameter access sheath has advantage over 9.5 Fr access sheath for this purpose as larger fragments can be retrieved. However, it should be noted that if ureter cannot be dilated with gentle maneuvers, then smaller access sheath should be used to prevent trauma to ureter.

Another way to address these stones is dusting these stones. The dusting is achieved with high frequency and low energy of Ho: YAG laser setting. The dusting setting is useful for relatively larger size of stone for which large number of fragment retrieval may increase operative time and hence amount of irrigation. Dusting setting is also useful in case of tight ureters when no access sheath is placed to avoid multiple passages across the narrow ureter which potentially increases the chances of ureteric injury and when a 9.5-Fr access sheath is placed as the size of fragment that can be retrieved is very small. However, it is to be noted that dusting may not be possible with hard stones like calcium oxalate mono-hydrate. The hard stones produce multiple fragments even with dusting setting which makes retrieval of fragments necessary. In such situations, patient should be placed with DJ stents to aid fragment passage and planned for second stage procedure for residual fragments after an interval.

C. Management of Small Stones in Lower Calyx

For treatment of lower calyceal stones thinner laser fiber (200 μm) should be used to facilitate lasing in lower calyces. The ideal settings should be for fragmentation. Once few fragments are created then stones can be basketted and placed into middle or upper calyces, where it can be lased easily without causing damage to deflection mechanism of flexible ureteroscope. Various baskets are available for commercial usage and are listed below (Table 13.5 and Fig. 13.11).

- NCircle™ (Cook Medical, Spencer, IN) is a tipless nitinol manipulator of length 115 cm and is available in various sizes (1.5, 2.2, 3 and 4.5 Fr). NCompass™ (Cook Medical, Spencer, IN) has 12 to 16 tightly weaved wires for removal of multiple stone fragments and is available as 1.7 and 2.4 Fr. Both of the above have a tipless design, cause very little damage to the papilla or urothelium and do not occupy much space upon opening (<1–2 cm when fully opened) and hence are useful in small compact calyces too.
- NForce™ (Cook Medical, Spencer, IN) is constructed of nitinol Delta Wire® and maintains the helical shape of the basket despite extreme torsion and hence effectively increases the radial force.
- Other baskets such as Parachute (Boston Scientific, MA), Lithocatch (Boston Scientific, MA) and Sur-Catch (Olympus,

PA) have more wires on the distal end of the basket and thus are reliable for removing multiple small fragments.

Two designs combine the safety and reliability of the graspers and baskets respectively. They can be specifically used for advancement over the stone and disengaging and removal of the stone.

- NGage™ (Cook Medical, Spencer, IN) is available as 1.7 and 2.2 Fr and has a patented triangular shape on opening. This basket can engage, reposition and has a superior ability to release the stone in comparison to multiwire nitinol baskets.
- Graspit™ (Boston Scientific) has a serrated wire edge that provides a secure grasp and helps in more effective stone retrieval or repositioning (2.6 and 3.2 Fr).

It is advisable to have separate flexible ureteroscope for treatment of lower calyceal stone in large volume centers. Newer flexible ureteroscope with preserved deflection mechanism may be used only for awkward lower calyceal stones and once the deflection has deteriorated it may be used for middle and

Table 13.5: List of baskets/retropulsion devices				
Model	Available size (Fr)	Available basket size (mm)	Length (cm)	Features
Dimension (Bard)	2.4, 3.0	10, 13, 16	115	Articulating four-wire, zero tip
Expand 212 (Bard)	3.0	11	90, 115	Articulating, 2-1-2-1, wire design filiform tip
Escape (Boston Scientific)	1.9	11, 15	90, 120	4-wire cage with channel for 200 micron laser fiber
Optiflex (Boston Scientific)	1.3	6, 7, 9, 11	90, 120	Rotates 360°, can entrap small fragments with preservation of vision
Zerotip (Boston Scientific)	1.9, 2.4, 3.0	12, 16	90, 120	Zero tip helps entrapment near parenchyma
NCircle (Cook Medical)	2.4	10, 20	115	Triangular shape allows very large wire mass, tipless mass
NForce (Cook Medical)	2.2, 3.2		115	3-wire
NGage (Cook Medical)	1.7, 2.2	8, 11	115	Allows repositioning

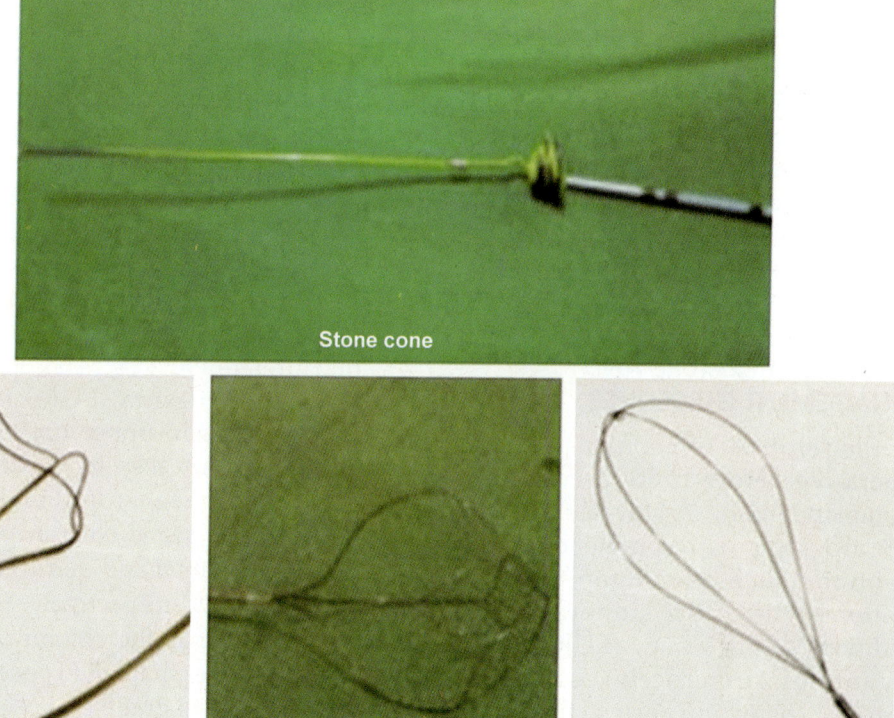

Fig. 13.11: Baskets and retropulsion devices

upper calyceal stones. This may result in better success rates in treatment of lower calyceal stones.

D. Management of Large Renal Stones and Staghorn Stones

The indication of flexible ureteroscopy in large renal stone and staghorn stone is in a patient with very high risk for percutaneous nephrolithotomy, e.g. patient with uncontrolled coagulopathies or patient in whom anti-coagulants cannot be discontinued for percutaneous nephrolithotomy. It should be noted that RIRS should be avoided in large infected stones if those stones can be managed with percutaneous nephrolithotomy. It is advisable to counsel all patients planned for RIRS for the need of prestenting and staged procedure in case of incomplete clearance, particularly in very large and staghorn stones where it is more likely to be required.

The irrigation flow of 20 ml/minute is sufficient for maintaining good vision in most of RIRS procedures. The laser setting during treatment of these stones should be dusting setting of high frequency and low energy as the fragments produced with lithotripsy of large stone are bulky in volume and it may not be possible to retrieve it with basket. After dusting of large stone, huge amount of dust is created and vision can be improved if large access sheath of 12 Fr is used for good continuous drainage. If vision is poor due to large dust created or if entire pelvicalyceal system gets coated with dust of stone, the procedure should be staged. Lasing in poor vision can be counterproductive as it may cause mucosal trauma, bleeding, perforation and intravasation leading to sepsis post-operatively. Ureter should be stented at end of procedure to facilitate drainage and passage of fragments and dust. Postoperatively, the

X-ray kidney ureter bladder of RIRS for large stone procedure may show entire pelvi-calyceal system coated with stone or diffuse radioopacity in entire pelvicalyceal system or multiple fragments in entire pelvicalyceal system. Later these patients will need radiological evaluation after interval and if significant residual stones are present in pelvi-calyceal system they may need second stage procedures.

REVIEW OF LITERATURE AND MANAGEMENT GUIDELINES

A preoperative noncontrast CT scan is imperative before ureteroscopy (grade C recommendation).[7] A contrast enhanced CT with urography is recommended in special situations such as congenital abnormal location or lie of the kidneys, obstructive conditions of the kidney (PUJO, obstructive megaureter, ureterocele), complex stone anatomy, prior surgeries, unusual body habitus and spinal dysraphisms.[8, 9]

Routine stenting before FURS is not recommended. Few studies have pointed towards higher success rates[10] for renal stones (67% versus 47%) and shorter operative time and lesser retreatment rates for stones less than 10 mm[11] and 5 mm.[12] Despite this association, AUA panel recommends against routine stenting as the benefit of higher success rates are superseded by the additional costs and the negative impact on the quality of life (evidence level grade B). Decompression with a DJ stent or PCN is advocated only in conditions of untreated infection and obstruction (evidence level grade C). Although RCTs have shown both to be equally effective,[13] the choice between DJ and PCN is usually the discretion of the treating urologist, and the factors to be considered are the clinical symptoms and their duration, presence of floating echogenic material/pus in the PCS, degree of dilatation of the calyces, the location of the stone and the proposed method of stone clearance. In a comparative study, Borofsky et al showed that mortality after FURS in the presence of active infection was significantly higher in those who underwent surgery without decompression (19.2%) as against those who underwent surgery after decom-pression (8.8%).[14]

For ureteral stones, FURS has more success rates and fewer procedures are needed in comparison to SWL.[15] For stones less than 10 mm, stone-free rates are superior for FURS than SWL in upper ureters (91% *vs* 75%) and mid ureters (94% *vs* 74%). For larger stones more than 10 mm, FURS has equivalent success rates in upper ureter (79% *vs* 74%) and better success in midureters (82% *vs* 67%). The mean number of procedures required for stone clearance for FURS and SWL in proximal and midureters are 1.01, 1.0 and 1.34, 1.29, respectively. In light of these reasons, URS is the recommendation for all ureteric stones that failed observation or MET (evidence level grade B). For patients who do not want URS, physicians can offer SWL with an understanding that it is a lesser morbid procedure with lower complications, albeit with lower success rates (evidence level grade B).

The upper ureteric stone should be managed with a flexible ureteroscope as the semirigid ureteroscopes have lesser success rates and more morbidity. Semirigid uretero-scopes are unable to accommodate the angulation of the prostate and iliac vessels, thereby increasing the chances of both ureteral injury and damage to the ureteroscope itself. Studies have shown that the flexible uretero-scopes have higher success rates and lower retreatment rates.[16–18]

The treatment algorithms of renal calculi are outlined below. For non-lower polar symptomatic renal stones less than 1 cm, EAU guidelines recommend SWL as the preferred option and FURS as an alternative option (evidence level grade B). The literature supporting this preference comes from the time period when Dornier HM3 was used in

SWL. Since then, lithotripters have become smaller for decreasing anesthetic requirements and flexible ureteroscopes have undergone a revolutionary change. Contemporary studies have suggested better stone clearance and lesser retreatment rates with ureteroscopy for stones less than 1 cm[19] than SWL. Although both SWL and FURS are less invasive than PCNL, FURS has reported more complications than SWL. With technological advancements, Global Ureteroscopy Study reported an overall complication rates of 3.5% with FURS with ureteral stricture (0.4%), sepsis (0.3%) and death (0.03%) occurring rarely.[20] All these factors taken together, recent literature tilts the balance in favor of FURS with an excellent safety profile, and stone-free rates and treatment efficiency better than SWL for small stones.

For stones between 1 and 2 cm, factors which negatively affect the success of SWL such as composition of stone (cystine, brushite), stone Hounsfield unit >1000 and skin to stone distance >10 cm may aid in better decision making between FURS and SWL.[21–23] Single sitting success rates are definitely higher with FURS, 90% for upper and middle calyceal stones and 80% for lower calyceal stones. Even better stone clearance rates can be achieved with mini PERC or micro PERC, although more randomized multicentric studies are required before advocating one modality over the other.

For stones more than 2 cm, both AUA and EAU guidelines recommend PCNL as the preferred option and recommend against SWL (evidence level grade C). PCNL results in better and more complete stone clearance, and this success is unaffected by stone location, density and composition. FURS typically requires multiple treatment sessions and longer operative time with the risk of sepsis. PCNL is invasive with more bleeding complications (6–7%)[24, 25] with blood transfusion requirement being 1–2%. With the advent of high power lasers, the operative times of FURS have significantly come down and the clinical impact is still not known. Although there are reports of treatment of even staghorn calculi safely with staged FURS, these come from high volume centers and more prospective studies are required before stretching the limits of FURS or incorporation into guidelines for management of high burden stones in the kidney.

For failures after SWL, ureteroscopy is an option and for failures after FURS, PCNL is an option (grade C recommendation). The remaining stone burden and the location should be considered in the decision making. A small significant fragment might as well be treated with FURS again and removing the fragment using a basket. Multiple fragments or a large remaining stone burden will mandate PCNL and stone clearance.

The lower pole stones continue to remain an Enigma for the following reasons. The inherent unfavorable anatomy due to the acute angle, long infundibular length and narrow infundibular width becomes challenging and the ureteroscope may not reach the stone in quite a few cases. In view of the dependent nature, the fragments may not pass spontaneously and mandates positioning and percussion techniques. The fragments may remain despite these adjunctive maneuvers and necessitate a second procedure. With the use of CT for checking residual fragments, these retained fragments may raise a medicolegal aspect for these fragments as well. A single procedure to maximally and safely clear the stone should be the aim for all renal stones, especially those of the lower pole.

For lower polar stones less than 10 mm, SWL or FURS should be offered as primary modality of treatment (evidence level grade C). Multiple prospective randomized controlled trials have established the equivalent success rates of both, the complications are more with FURS and quality of life outcomes are better with SWL.[26] Factors which negatively affect the success of SWL such as composition of stone (cystine, brushite), stone Hounsfield unit >1000, skin to stone distance >10 cm and unfavorable anatomy (narrow infundibulopelvic angle, narrow infundibulum and long calyx) may become vital in a given case.[21–23] Repositioning of these small stones into upper calyx, removal of generated fragments and usage of access sheath further improves the safety and success of FURS.[27, 28]

PCNL is currently the treatment of choice for uncomplicated lower polar stones of size more than 2 cm in view of higher single treatment success rates, albeit with higher complications (evidence level grade B).[26] The specific concerns of ureteroscopy are that the stones may not be reachable during the procedure, inability to relocate the large stones into favorable calyx, *in situ* dusting leading to many fragments and considerable amount of dust which can settle down in the dependent lower calyx and the damage to the ureteroscope during lower polar laser usage. Although these risk exist during small stone treatment as well, but the sheer long operative time in a flexed position may create a considerable damage to the ureteroscope. Hence, for larger stone burden, PCNL should be the primary treating modality.

SPECIAL SITUATIONS

Pediatric Population

Pediatric ureteroscopy was first described by Ritchey et al in 1998. The concerns of large size of the instruments, fragile pediatric ureters and non-availability of smaller accessory instruments impeded the growth of pediatric ureteroscopy. It took a decade for further development in the field of pediatric FURS, especially with the advent of smaller shaft ureteroscopes and improved accessories. widespread availability of lasers paved the way for modern day ureteroscopies in children with technical ease.

Pediatric ureters are more pliable than the adult ureters and hence are technically easier to dilate before ureteroscopy. Single stage

procedures are possible and safer for stones smaller than 2 cm, FURS is definitely an option for stones more than 2 cm, the success rates drastically go down, and passage of fragments in children is something we cannot depend upon, especially post-procedure.

Horseshoe Kidneys

The most common complication of horseshoe kidneys is renal stones with an incidence of up to 20–40%. Impaired urinary drainage with consequent stasis and infection predisposes to stone formation in horseshoe kidneys. Endourological management of these calculi are the accepted gold standard, but the decision and choice of a particular endourological procedure requires careful evaluation and judicious planning.

FURS is an attractive option for smaller stone burden, albeit at slightly lower success rates (75–80%).[29] The proposed reasons for lower success rates are: Ureteral access related issues, decreased maneuverability due to bending of the scope at the anteriorly displaced PUJ, improper case selection with larger stone burden and impaired drainage due to anatomical factors. But the FURS had a distinct advantage in obese patients, in patients with bleeding diathesis and those with poor cardiopulmonary status who could not tolerate a prone position or laparoscopic procedure.

Ectopic Kidneys

In ectopic kidneys, variation in ureteral insertion, tortuosities and angulations in the ureter are the major concerns with FURS. Placement of a ureteral access sheath is invaluable as it straightens the ureter and allows easy passage of the ureteroscope and egress of the fluid and fragments and helps with faster clearance. Miniaturization of the scopes, availability of slender and powerful lasers and smaller accessories like the nitinol baskets have improved our success rates tremendously over yesteryears.

The introduction of digital chip on tip flexible ureteroscopes is big breakthrough for flexible ureteroscopy. A study comparing Flex-XC (Karl Storz GMBH and Co. KG-Tuttlingen) which is digital flexible ureteroscope and Flex-X2 (Karl Storz GMBH and Co. KG-Tuttlingen) showed that Flex-XC has better vision, improved color resolution and better visualization of upper tracts, better deflection and light weight compared to Flex-X2.[30] The Flex-XC had better vision in both hemorrhagic field as well as clear field. The flow of irrigation was also better with Flex-XC with or without accessories in instrument channels. This study compared these instruments *in vitro* as well as *in vivo* condition in porcine models.[30]

Multescu et al compared digital and fiberoptic flexible ureteroscope suggested that digital flexible ureteroscopes have better vision and maneuverability but it has limitation due to bigger shaft in case of narrow infundibulum.[31]

Further advancements of reusable digital flexible ureteroscope led to single use digital flexible ureteroscope. A study by Dale et al comparing LithoVue™, a single use digital flexible ureteroscope (Boston Scientific—Marlborough, MA) with Flex-XC, a reusable digital ureteroscope (Karl Storz GMBH and Co. KG-Tuttlingen) and COBRA, a reusable fiberoptic ureteroscope (Richard Wolf GMBH Knittlingen, Germany) showed LithoVue™ had largest field of vision, excellent vision and depth of image. LithoVue™ maintained full range of deflection despite instruments in working channel compared to other two which did not LithoVue™ and Flex-XC had similar flow rates without instrument in working channel but LithoVue™ had better flow with instrument in working channel. COBRA has separate irrigation channel which gives preserved flow rates despite instruments in working channels.[32]

Another prospective study comparing LithoVue™ and fiberoptic flexible ureteroscope suggested that LithoVue™ is associated with lesser scope failure rates and decreased procedural and operating room time with LithoVue™.[33] However, the authors state that the findings need to be substantiated with further studies.

A study of economic implications of disposable versus reusable digital flexible ureteroscope suggest that disposable flexible ureteroscopes are economical in set ups with low volume of flexible ureteroscopy per year, whereas for large volume centers, reusable ureteroscopes are more economical.[34]

Robotic platform for performing flexible ureteroscopy has been introduced. Roboflex Avicenna is a robotic platform for flexible ureteroscopy. Initial studies with Roboflex[35] suggested that all flexible ureteroscopies were successful without conversion to manual ureteroscopy. There were no intraoperative complications. A study comparing flexible ureteroscopy with or without Roboflex Avicenna platform demonstrated comparable outcome with better comfort for operating surgeon.[36]

High fidelity ureteroscopy trainers such as URS trainer (Ideal Anatomic Modelling, Holt, Michigan, USA) are available in select centers. Virtual reality models are also available for endourological procedures and have had a profound effect in reducing the learning curve associated with this procedure in particular.[37]

As FURS continues to be more and more increasingly used and becoming widely available, it is important to develop a structured, effective and reproducible way to disseminate surgical techniques to junior colleagues. Simulators result in a more rapid learning and acquiring of skills in FURS than conventional training methods. FURS simulators are very promising for training, and have the advantage of minimizing the need to learn procedures and time spent on patients.[38]

References

1. Smith AD, Preminger G, Badlani G, Kavoussi LR. Smith's Textbook of Endourology: Flexible fiber-optic ureteropyeloscopy: Edition 2nd, Volume 1st.

2. Marshall VF. Fiberoptics in urology. J Urol 1964; 91:110–14.

3. Tagaki T, Go T, Takayasu H, et al. A small caliber fiberscope for the visualization of the urinary tract, biliary tract and spinal canal. Surgery 1968;64: 1033–38.

4. Pietrow PK, Auge BK, Delvecchio FC, et al. Techniques to maximize flexible ureteroscope longevity. Urology 2002;60(5):784–88.

5. Culkin DJ, Exaire EJ, Green D, et al. Anticoagulation and antiplatelet therapy in urological practice: ICUD/AUA review paper. J Urol 2014 Oct; 192(4):1026–34.

6. Moses Elhilali MM, Badaan S, Ibrahim A, Andonian S. Use of the Moses Technology to Improve Holmium Laser Lithotripsy Outcomes: A Preclinical Study. Journal of Endourology. 2017 Jun 1.

7. Fulgham PF, Assimos DG, Pearle MS, et al. Clinical effectiveness protocols for imaging in the management of ureteral calculous disease: AUA technology assessment. J Urol 2013;189:1230.

8. Patel U, Walkden RM, Ghani KR, et al. Three-dimensional CT pyelography for planning of percutaneous nephrostolithotomy: accuracy of stone measurement, stone depiction and pelvicalyceal reconstruction. Eur Radiol 2009; 19: 1280.

9. Thiruchelvam N, Mostafid H, Ubhayakar G. Planning percutaneous nephrolithotomy using multidetector computed tomography urography, multiplanar reconstruction and three-dimensional reformatting. BJU Int 2005;95:1280.

10. Rubenstein RA, Zhao LC, Loeb S, et al. Prestenting improves ureteroscopic stone-free rates. J Endourol 2007;21:1277.

11. Chu L, Farris CA, Corcoran AT, et al. Preoperative stent placement decreases cost of ureteroscopy. Urology 2011;78:309.

12. Netsch C, Knipper S, Bach T, et al. Impact of preoperative ureteral stenting on stone-free rates of ureteroscopy for nephroureterolithiasis: a matched-paired analysis of 286 patients. Urology 2012;80:1214.

13. Pearle MS, Pierce HL, Miller GL, et al. Optimal method of urgent decompression of the collecting system for obstruction and infection due to ureteral calculi. J Urol 1998;160:1260.

14. Borofsky MS, Walter D, Shah O, et al. Surgical decompression is associated with decreased mortality in patients with sepsis and ureteral calculi. J Urol 2013;189:946.

15. Preminger GM, Tiselius HG, Assimos DG, et al. 2007 guideline for the management of ureteral calculi. J Urol 2007;178:2418.

16. Cohen J, Cohen S, Grasso M. Ureteropyeloscopic treatment of large, complex intrarenal and proximal ureteral calculi. BJU Int 2013;111:E127.

17. Hyams E, Monga M, Pearle MS, et al. A prospective, multi-institutional study of flexible ureteroscopy for proximal ureteral stones smaller than 2 cm. J Urol 2015;193:165.

18. Perez Castro E, Osther PJ, Jinga V, et al. Differences in ureteroscopic stone treatment and outcomes for distal, mid-proximal, or multiple ureteral locations: the Clinical Research Office of the Endourological Society ureteroscopy global study. Eur Urol 2014; 66:102.

19. Matlaga BR, Jansen JP, Meckley LM, et al. Treatment of ureteral and renal stones: a systematic review and meta-analysis of randomized, controlled trials. J Urol 2012;188:130.

20. De La Rosette J, Denstedt J, Geavlete P, Keeley F, Matsuda T, Pearle M, Preminger G, Traxer O, CROES URS study group. The clinical research office of the endourological society ureteroscopy global study: indications, complications, and outcomes in 11,885 patients. Journal of Endourology 2014 Feb 1;28(2):131–9.

21. Pareek G, Hedican SP, Lee FT JR, et al. Shock wave lithotripsy success determined by skin-to-stone distance on computed tomography. Urology. 2005;66:941.

22. Joseph P, Mandal AK, Singh SK, et al. Computerized tomography attenuation value of renal calculus: can it predict successful fragmentation of the calculus by extracorporeal shock wave lithotripsy? A preliminary study. J Urol 2002;167:1968.

23. Perks AE, Schuler TD, Lee J, et al. Stone attenuation and skin-to-stone distance on computed tomography predicts for stone fragmentation by shock wave lithotripsy. Urology 2008;72:765.

24. de la Rosette J, Assimos D, Desai M, et al. The Clinical Research Office of the Endourological Society Percutaneous Nephrolithotomy Global Study: indications, complications, and outcomes in 5,803 patients. J Endourol 2011;25:11.

25. Seitz C, Desai M, Hacker A, et al. Incidence, prevention, and management of complications following percutaneous nephrolitholapaxy. Eur Urol 2012;61:146.

26. Pearle MS, Lingeman JE, Leveillee R, et al. Prospective, randomized trial comparing shock wave lithotripsy and ureteroscopy for lower pole calyceal calculi 1 cm or less. J Urol 2005;173:2005.

27. Schuster TG, Hollenbeck BK, Faerber GJ, et al. Ureteroscopic treatment of lower pole calculi: comparison of lithotripsy *in situ* and after displacement. J Urol 2002;168:43.

28. L'esperance JO, Ekeruo WO, Scales CD Jr, et al. Effect of ureteral access sheath on stone-free rates in patients undergoing ureteoscopic management of renal calculi. Urology 2005;66:252.

29. Weizer AZ, Springhart WP, Ekeruo WO, Matlaga BR, Tan YH, Assimos DG, Preminger GM. Ureteroscopic management of renal calculi in anomalous kidneys. Urology 2005 Feb 28;65(2): 265–69.

30. Lusch A1, Abdelshehid C, Hidas G, et al. *In vitro* and *in vivo* comparison of optics and performance of a distal sensor ureteroscope versus a standard fiberoptic ureteroscope. J Endourol 2013 Jul;27(7): 896–902.

31. Multescu R, Geavlete B, Georgescu D, Geavlete P. Conventional fiberoptic flexible ureteroscope versus fourth generation digital flexible uretero-scope: a critical comparison. J Endourol 2010 Jan;24(1):17–21.

32. Dale J, Kaplan AG, Radvak D, et al. Evaluation of a Novel Single Use Flexible Ureteroscope. Dale J1, Kaplan AG1, Radvak D2, et al.

33. Usawachintachit M, Isaacson DS, Taguchi K, et al. A Prospective Case-Control Study Comparing LithoVue, a Single-Use, Flexible Disposable Ureteroscope, with Flexible, Reusable Fiber-Optic Ureteroscopes.J Endourol 2017 May;31(5):468–75.

34. Martin CJ, McAdams SB, Abdul-Muhsin H. The Economic Implications of a Reusable Flexible Digital Ureteroscope: A Cost-Benefit Analysis. J Urol 2017 Mar;197(3 Pt 1):730–35.

35. Desai MM, Grover R, Aron M, et al. Robotic flexible ureteroscopy for renal calculi: initial clinical experience. J Urol 2011 Aug;186(2):563–68.

36. Geavlete P, Saglam R, Georgescu D, et al. Robotic Flexible Ureteroscopy Versus Classic Flexible Ureteroscopy in Renal Stones: the Initial Romanian Experience. Chirurgia (Bucur). 2016 Jul-Aug; 111(4):326–29.

37. Dolmans VE, Schout BM, de Beer NA, Bemelmans BL, Scherpbier AJ, Hendrikx AJ. The virtual reality endourologic simulator is realistic and useful for educational purposes. J Endourol 2009;23:1175–81.

38. Seitz C, Fajkovic H. Training in ureteroscopy for urolithiasis. Arab Journal of Urology 2014;12(1): 42–48.

Index